Sociocultural Examinations of Sports Concussions

Sport's "concussion crisis" has been characterized by controversial scientific discoveries, athlete suicides, and high-profile lawsuits involving professional sports leagues, while provoking widespread media coverage, changes to game rules, and debate about the future of many popular sports. *Sociocultural Examinations of Sports Concussions* is the first edited collection to bring together multiple sociocultural perspectives on sports concussion that interrogate the social, economic, political, and historical forces shaping the cultural impacts of these injuries.

Each of the ten chapters moves beyond biomedical or neuroscientific paradigms to critically examine a specific intersection of sociocultural factors influencing public perceptions about concussion or athlete experiences of brain injury. These include analyses of media and advertising, medical treatment and diagnostic protocols, gender and masculinity, developments in equipment and scientific models, economics and labor politics, understandings of trauma and recovery, public health philosophies, and disciplinary differences in framing the ontologies of concussion.

Drawing from a wide range of theoretical and methodological approaches, *Sociocultural Examinations of Sports Concussions* offers a diverse set of analyses examining brain injuries as cultural and embodied phenomena affecting more than just athletes' brains, but also embedded within and (re)shaping meanings, identities, and social contexts. It is valuable reading for graduate students and researchers interested in the experience and treatment of sports concussion, sports sociology, and sports technology.

Matt Ventresca is a postdoctoral associate in the Faculty of Kinesiology at the University of Calgary (Alberta, Canada), where he is affiliated with the Integrated Concussion Research Program. Dr. Ventresca previously completed his PhD at Queen's University and was a postdoctoral fellow in the School of History and Sociology at the Georgia Institute of Technology (USA). Matt's research concerns the intersections of social inequalities, media, and science in the contexts of sport and health. His current work focuses on the sociocultural implications of traumatic brain injuries (TBI) in sports contexts, centering, specifically, on the processes through which knowledge about TBI gets produced through media representations and scientific research practices. Matt studies the sociocultural dimensions of pain and injury in sports more broadly, as well as the promotional cultures surrounding popular men's health initiatives.

Mary G. McDonald is the Homer C. Rice Chair in Sports and Society in the School of History and Sociology at the Georgia Institute of Technology (USA). A past president of the North American Society for the Sociology of Sport, Professor McDonald's research focuses on American culture and sport including issues of inequality as related to gender, race, class, and sexuality. She recently has begun to expand this analysis by engaging science and technology studies theories and methods to critically investigate sporting technologies. As Homer C. Rice Chair, she is directing the Ivan Allen College of Liberal Arts initiative, the Sports, Society, and Technology Program.

Routledge Research in Sport and Exercise Science

The *Routledge Research in Sport and Exercise Science* series is a showcase for cutting-edge research from across the sport and exercise sciences, including physiology, psychology, biomechanics, motor control, physical activity and health, and every core sub-discipline. Featuring the work of established and emerging scientists and practitioners from around the world, and covering the theoretical, investigative and applied dimensions of sport and exercise, this series is an important channel for new and ground-breaking research in the human movement sciences.

Available in this series:

Modelling and Simulation in Sport and Exercise
Edited by Arnold Baca and Jürgen Perl

The Exercising Female
Science and Application
Edited by Jacky J. Forsyth and Claire-Marie Roberts

Genetics and the Psychology of Motor Performance
Sigal Ben-Zaken, Veronique Richard, Gershon Tenenbaum

Psychological Aspects of Sport-Related Concussions
Edited by Gordon A. Bloom and Jeffrey G. Caron

Human Fatigue
Evolution, Health and Disease
Frank Marino

Sociocultural Examinations of Sports Concussions
Edited by Matt Ventresca and Mary G. McDonald

For more information about this series, please visit: www.routledge.com/sport/series/RRSES

Sociocultural Examinations of Sports Concussions

Edited by Matt Ventresca and
Mary G. McDonald

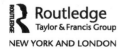

NEW YORK AND LONDON

First published 2020
by Routledge
52 Vanderbilt Avenue, New York, NY 10017

and by Routledge
2 Park Square, Milton Park, Abingdon, Oxon, OX14 4RN

Routledge is an imprint of the Taylor & Francis Group, an informa business

First issued in paperback 2021

Library of Congress Cataloging-in-Publication Data
Names: Ventresca, Matt, editor.
Title: Sociocultural examinations of sports concussions/
    edited by Matt Ventresca and Mary G. McDonald.
Description: New York : Routledge, 2019. | Series: Routledge
    research in sport and exercise science | Includes bibliographical
    references and index.
Identifiers: LCCN 2019033638 (print) | LCCN 2019033639
    (ebook) | ISBN 9780367134501 (hardcover) | ISBN
    9780429028175 (ebook)
Subjects: LCSH: Brain–Concussions. | Sports injuries–Psychological
    aspects. | Sports–Sociological aspects. | Sports and state.
Classification: LCC RC394.C7 S63 2019 (print) | LCC RC394.C7
    (ebook) | DDC 617.4/81044–dc23
LC record available at https://lccn.loc.gov/2019033638
LC ebook record available at https://lccn.loc.gov/2019033639

ISBN: 978-0-367-13450-1 (hbk)
ISBN: 978-1-03-208532-6 (pbk)
ISBN: 978-0-429-02817-5 (ebk)

Typeset in Galliard
by Apex CoVantage, LLC

Contents

PART III
The Politics of Trauma, Experience, and Research 95

Figure

Contributors

Kathleen Bachynski is Assistant Professor of Public Health, Muhlenberg College, USA.

Sean Brayton is Associate Professor in the Department of Kinesiology and Physical Education, in Faculty of Arts and Science at the University of Lethbridge, Canada.

William Bridel is Assistant Professor in the Faculty of Kinesiology, University of Calgary, Canada.

Daniel S. Goldberg is Core Faculty, Center for Bioethics and Humanities and Associate Professor in the Department of Family Medicine (CU School of Medicine) and the Department of Epidemiology (CO School of Public Health) at the University of Colorado Anschutz Medical Campus.

Michelle T. Helstein is Associate Professor in the Department of Kinesiology and Physical Education in the Faculty of Arts and Science at the University of Lethbridge, Canada.

Kathryn Henne holds the Canada Research Chair in Biogovernance, Law and Society at the University of Waterloo, where she is a fellow of the Balsillie School of International Affairs. She is also Associate Professor at RegNet, the School of Regulation and Global Governance at the Australian National University.

Danika Kelly is a graduate student in the Faculty of Kinesiology, University of Calgary, Canada.

Dominic Malcolm is Reader in the Sociology of Sport, Loughborough University, UK.

Mary G. McDonald is Homer C. Rice Chair of Sports and Society, and Professor in the School of History and Sociology at the Georgia Institute of Technology, USA.

Daniel R. Morrison is Assistant Professor of Sociology, Abilene Christian University, USA.

Kathryn Schneider is Associate Professor in the Faculty of Kinesiology & Sport Injury Prevention Research Centre (SIPRC), University of Calgary, Canada.

Cathy van Ingen is Associate Professor in the Department of Kinesiology at Brock University, Canada.

Matt Ventresca is a Postdoctoral Associate in the Faculty of Kinesiology, University of Calgary, Canada.

Kevin Viliunas is an undergraduate student in the Faculty of Kinesiology, University of Calgary, Canada.

Acknowledgments

The works collected in this anthology came out of a three-day workshop hosted at the Georgia Institute of Technology in March 2018. We would like to thank those who attended this workshop for their enthusiastic participation in discussions that shaped the content of this book. This includes, of course, our fabulous contributors, whose hard work is reflected in the insightful arguments that comprise this collection. Our initial goal of bringing together a group of sociocultural scholars interested in sport-related brain injury would simply not have been conceivable without these authors' previous contributions to the critical analysis of this issue. We would also like to acknowledge the support of the School of History and Sociology at the Georgia Institute of Technology, as well as the Faculty of Kinesiology and Integrated Concussion Research Program at the University of Calgary. Financial support for the anthology comes from funds provided through the Homer C. Rice Chair in Sports and Society and the Sports, Society, and Technology Program at the Georgia Institute of Technology. Our sincerest thanks go to David Varley, Megan Smith, and our team at Routledge for their encouragement and professional guidance around the completion of this project.

Part I
Introduction

1 Forces of Impact

Critically Examining Sport's "Concussion Crises"

Matt Ventresca and Mary G. McDonald

As concern about traumatic brain injury (TBI) in sports has intensified over the past three decades, it has become strikingly ordinary to encounter declarations about how the contemporary sports world is in the throes of a "concussion crisis." Estimates for the number of concussions sustained in sports contexts per year vary widely. The most commonly cited statistics from the Center for Disease Control (CDC) specify an extremely wide range, approximating that somewhere between 1.6 and 3.8 million concussions occur annually in the United States (Harmon et al. 2013). Even without more precise injury rates, descriptions of the prevalence of concussion in sports as a "national obsession" (Cantu and Hyman 2012), "the number one contemporary sports issue" (Reed 2017), and a "silent epidemic" (Carroll and Rosner 2012) speak to the perceived urgency and severity of this "crisis." The apparent magnitude of the problem is further reflected in the sheer variety of developments connected to, and emerging from, sport's "concussion crises."

National and international research programs, as well as scholarly organizations dedicated to the scientific study of concussion, have been founded. Professional and amateur sports organizations have approved rule changes to protect athletes from brain trauma. Companies have invested millions into developing technologies related to the diagnosis and prevention of concussion, from protective equipment and digital impact sensors to pharmaceutical treatments and nutritional supplements. Governments have enacted legislation to support more comprehensive sideline medical care for concussed athletes. Multi-million-dollar concussion lawsuits have been brought against high-profile sports organizations such as the National Football League (NFL), the National Hockey League (NHL), and the National Collegiate Athletic Association (NCAA). News stories about concussion have become an everyday part of the sports media landscape. A previously obscure neurodegenerative disease, chronic traumatic encephalopathy (CTE), has become a commonly discussed topic among athletes, sports commentators, and fans. Hollywood mega-star Will Smith even played a neuropathologist in a feature film about the discovery of CTE in the brain of an NFL player.

The "concussion crisis" has notably also infiltrated the realm of American politics. In 2014, then U.S. President Barack Obama hosted the "Healthy Kids and Safe Sports Concussion Summit," a gathering which brought together over 200 sports officials, scientists, clinicians, coaches, parents, and young athletes in conversation about how to best address brain injuries in youth sports. The summit was a venue for sharing the latest scientific breakthroughs and discussing opportunities for better diagnosis and treatment, but Obama also made comments highlighting the cultural dimensions of concussion. Obama asserted, "We have to change a culture that says, 'you suck it up and play through a brain injury'. The president continued, "It doesn't make you weak" to report a concussion, "it means you're strong" (Diamond 2014).

Just over two years later, at an October campaign rally in Lakeland, Florida, soon-to-be President Donald J. Trump noticed a woman in the audience had fainted due to the extremely hot weather conditions. When the woman returned to the rally after receiving medical attention, Trump praised her resilience, joking, "See we don't go by these new and very much softer NFL rules. . . . Concussion? Uh oh, got a little ding on the head, no, no you can't play for the rest of the season. Our people are tough!" (Guarino 2016). Trump's comments are representative of widespread backlash to rule changes made in the interest of improving athlete health and safety, particularly in the hyper-masculine collision sport of gridiron football. Yet, importantly, Trump's remarks drew from a larger, ongoing analogy in which the NFL, its predominately African American playing force, and football culture, more broadly, were continuous targets of derision. Thomas Oates (2017, 169) explains how Trump connected football's apparent symbolic expressions of "hegemonic masculinity to a national decline, reframing a debate about individual safety as a defense of America's future." Contrary to Obama's call for action to address brain injury in youth sports, Trump's analogy depicts concerns about concussion as representative of a collective "softening" of American culture and antithetical to his brand of white masculine populism.

Scholars have identified that "the problem" of concussion is almost exclusively conceptualized through a biomedical or neuroscientific lens, where the extent of the injury is defined according to impairments across biological systems (Malcolm 2017; Ventresca 2019). Yet such contrasting comments from two American presidents vividly illustrate how the materiality of sports concussions is intertwined with cultural norms and ideologies. This edited collection, *Sociocultural Examinations of Sports Concussions*, seeks to critically engage such entanglements of the biological and the cultural. Derived from a research symposium held in March 2018 at the Georgia Institute of Technology, this interdisciplinary anthology brings together critical analyses of the cultural implications of brain injuries in sports investigated through relevant histories, controversies, experiences, and knowledge formations.

The chapters that make up this book move beyond analyses of concussion conducted through biomedical or neuroscientific lenses to interrogate the social, economic, political, and historical forces shaping the cultural impact of these injuries. Each of the following nine chapters critically examines a specific intersection of sociocultural factors influencing public perceptions about concussion or athlete experiences of brain injury, including media and advertising, medical treatment and diagnostic protocols, gender and masculinity, developments in equipment and changing scientific paradigms, economics and labor politics, understandings of trauma and recovery, and public health philosophies. Drawing from a wide range of theoretical and methodological approaches that characterize the social sciences and humanities, *Sociocultural Examinations of Sports Concussions* offers a diverse set of analyses examining brain injuries as *cultural and material* phenomena affecting more than just an athlete's brain, but also embedded within and (re)shaping meanings, identities, and social contexts.

Concussion and the Sociological Imagination

The analytical focus of this anthology is first indebted to the tradition of critical scholarship including C. Wright Mills' (1959) arguments about the importance of developing a *sociological imagination*. The sociological imagination involves tracing connections between patterns in individual lives and those in society, noticing how personal biographies are shaped by larger socio-historical contexts. The sociological imagination is, therefore, crucially distinct from medical or psychological perspectives, because it moves beyond the study of individual physiology or behavior and instead examines how events, experiences, and ideas are influenced by societal trends. As such, the sociological imagination encompasses three components: historical, comparative, and critical analyses.

Historical examinations allow for mapping change over time and facilitating better understandings of contemporary events by situating them in historical contexts. Comparative analysis enables assessing phenomena across different societies, (sub)cultures, and social environments, thus cultivating an openness to possibilities and ideas beyond dominant ways of thinking. Critical scrutiny requires recognizing how personal problems and societal issues are linked to power imbalances and social inequalities. Thus, critical analysis encourages the questioning of taken-for-granted assumptions about how the world works, while supporting societal improvements and movements toward social change.

The ethos offered via the sociological imagination has been vigorously taken up by scholars demonstrating how sports are cultural practices influenced by, and influencing, the larger societies in which they take place. Sports Studies scholars have, for decades, illustrated how sports are sites of ongoing social and political struggles over meaning, identities, resources, and power (Coakley 2017). These research directions have cultivated insight into how athletic bodies are enactments of beliefs and values about gender, race, social class, sexuality, (dis)ability, and nationhood (McDonald and Birrell 1999). Such analyses have especially contributed to scholarly work concerning sport-related pain and injury that examines how athletes experience and interpret pain, as well as how athletes construct identities through the management (and often disavowal) of pain and injury (Young 2004; Roderick 1998). This research has additionally raised questions about tensions between the unquestioned status of sports as "healthy" activities and the lived experiences of pain and injury, while also interrogating the governance of sports medicine and the discipline's often-conflicting goals of improving athlete health and enabling sport performance (Safai 2003; Theberge 2008).

Sociocultural Examinations of Sports Concussions is particularly indebted to these perspectives generated by Sport Studies scholars. The anthology also emerges with a growing body of related scholarship, especially evident from 2012 onwards, which draws from social sciences and humanities theories and methods to analyze concussion in sports contexts. While it would be impossible to fairly or exhaustively characterize this research, this scholarship's commitments to more deeply explore complex TBI assemblages are also evident in scholars' various engagements with historical, comparative, and critical sensitivities. A few examples are illustrative of this analytical commitment.

For example, Emily Harrison's (2014) investigation of "football's first concussion crisis," suggests that the recent emphasis on brain injuries is hardly new as extensive medical concern about head and brain injuries among US college football players existed in the late nineteenth and early twentieth centuries. As can be seen today, powerful community leaders sought to intervene to make sure that the sport was considered "safe enough" to ensure its long-term viability. This examination helps to contextualize a much longer process whereby brain and bodily health concerns in sports, particularly collision and contact sports, are often downplayed or brushed aside (see also Bachynski this volume). Stephen Casper (2018a, 2018b) has indeed illuminated how neuroscientific research directions around brain injury have historically shaped, but also been shaped by, cultural debates about the safety of collision sports such as boxing and football.

The last three decades have seen rapid growth in media content about concussion across news articles, sports broadcasts, film, social media posts, and podcasts, helping to raise public awareness; although some coverage has been framed in individualistic or sensationalistic ways, the latter of which, some scholars suggest, helps to overstate risks and perpetuate a culture of fear around the dangers of brain injury (Kuhn et al. 2017; Stewart et al. 2019). And yet, investigative reports, have shed light on unethical and dishonest practices undertaken by several sports organizations in the interests of maintaining athlete productivity and in avoiding legal responsibility for athlete well-being (e.g., Fainaru-Wada and Fainaru 2013). Scholars have investigated the intricacies of these sometimes contradictory media discourses, through which journalists disseminate information about advancements in concussion science while also providing unsettling accounts of athletes' experiences living in the aftermath of brain injury (Bell et al. 2019; Furness 2016; Ventresca 2019) and describing athletes' attempts to protect their own health (Anderson and Kian 2012; McGannon et al. 2013; Cassilo and Sanderson 2016). Ventresca's (2019) comparative analysis illustrates how competing media discourses too often privilege the illusion of scientific conclusiveness over athlete testimony in debates about collision sports' often violent effects. Researchers have also analyzed how information about TBI gets shared across social media, emphasizing the limitations of these platforms for disseminating accurate and relevant information about complex topics (Hull and Schmittel 2014). These examples demonstrate the contested character of cultural knowledge formations as well as the agenda-setting power of the media to socially construct meanings of concussions, often in reductive ways.

Research empirically examining lived experiences of concussion has largely critiqued the influence of social norms and expectations in shaping how athletes interpret and react to their injuries. Nikolaus Dean's (2019) autoethnography is a case in point as he describes his tumultuous experience of concussion and struggles with the ruptures between his embodied, injured reality and his desire to recapture his self-concept of a healthy, able-bodied athlete dedicated to broader sports values of self-sacrifice and determination (see also Cassilo and Sanderson 2018; Bridel et al. this volume). The linkage between masculinity and sporting norms helps to partially explain why some athletes celebrate "playing hurt" while taking an irreverent attitude toward concussion that downplays the severity of these injuries (Liston et al. 2018). Boneau et al. (2018) further implicate larger social processes at play by documenting how parents too often venerate family identities and community belonging as reasons for encouraging their children to play middle school football despite the potential risks to their boys' health and well-being.

Given the financial and legal stakes tied to developments in TBI science and policy, scholars have scrutinized what they view as industry-friendly framings of concussion debates and conflicts of interest in the funding of brain injury research. The NFL is a leader in this regard, using strategies that cast doubt on the existing science, thus obscuring any potential liability regarding player injuries (Goldberg 2012; also see Goldberg this volume). Brayton and colleagues (2019; see also Brayton and Helstein in this volume) also resist depoliticized readings of the collective fallout of concussion in professional sport, connecting medical debates about athletes' brain health with racialized labor struggles in the NFL and NHL. Malcolm (2017) further outlines the broader privileging of biomedical practitioners and protocols in TBI management and how the dominance of such approaches glosses over that concussion is foundationally a *social*, rather than a medical, problem (see also Morrison in this volume). Hardes (2017) and Ventresca (2020) similarly critique the primacy of neuroscience as a dominant knowledge paradigm in research and legal proceedings concerning concussion (see also Ventresca in this volume). However, Morrison and Casper (2016) question the relentless public focus on CTE in the NFL and highlight the lack of attention given to brain injuries sustained by victims of intimate partner violence (see also van Ingen in this volume). Morrison and Casper (2016) argue that the inflated concern about CTE among football players at the same time erases the embodied consequences of football experiences including by men who are also implicated in violence against women.

While hardly an exhaustive account, collectively this brief review addition-ally demonstrates that concussions are not simply physiological injuries but material sites of social meaning and political import. Such critical inquiries into the politics of concussion knowledge, embodiment, representations, and the "social arrangements of medical care" in sport environments (Roderick 2006, 24) are interconnected with broader investigations into the socio-historical processes shaping developments in biomedicine, scientific research, and technological innovations (Foucault 1973; Haraway 1997; Jasanoff 2005). Of particular relevance here are recent critical studies of neurosci-ence detailing how advancements in neuroimaging have facilitated new forms of human subjectivity and ways of thinking about brain function (Rose and Abi-Rached 2013; Dumit 2004; Pitts-Taylor 2016).

Among legitimate fears of biological determinism and neuroreductionism, which reduce humans to products of neural activity or brain chemistry, "the neurosciences are embracing a fundamentally social concept of the brain" (Pitts-Taylor 2016, 3). Feminists are at the forefront of such theorizing, examining "not merely the influence of culture on neurobiology but also the immanent multiplicity of neural matter itself, its refusal to be fully predictable" (Pitts-Taylor 2016, 10). Applied to sports settings, concussions should thus be conceived as material-semiotic phenomena (Ventresca 2019). Sociocultural analysis of concussion, then, does not exclusively pertain to the realm of "cul-ture" and "society," but rather can interrogate complex inter-actions (Barad 2007) among and between material "things" (brains, bodies, technologies, etc.) and "ideas" (scientific knowledge, social norms) through which brain injuries occur and are experienced.

Notes on Terminology

A central aim of this anthology is to help shape future scholarly and popu-lar discussion about sport's "concussion crisis." Part of this process requires interrogating the enduring use of the term "crisis" to characterize the extent of the problem. We recognize that crises don't just "happen" as an objective condition of reality but are actively *constructed* through discourses identifying and constituting the severity of problems (Hay 1996). Although use of the word "crisis" in the context of concussion unambiguously denotes times of immense difficulty or trouble for sport, the precise conditions of the "concus-sion crisis"—how serious is the threat? When did it start? Who is in peril? What is at stake?—remain decidedly less clear. Brain injuries are indeed troubling to important networks of suffering athletes, teammates, families, sport organi-zations, advertisers, medical personnel, fans, researchers, and media produc-ers (to mention but a few). Yet each of these stakeholder groups encounter distinct challenges—and possibilities—related to the problem of concussions that are contingent on socio-historical processes and varying conceptions of the nature of this "crisis." We therefore use the plural "crises" (rather than the popularly used and singular "crisis") in the title of this introduction to this collection to signify the multiple factors and contingencies contributing to (and detracting from) the sense of urgency around sports TBI. While recognizing the constructedness of these multiple "crises," however, we also embrace how discourses of crisis facilitate moments of possible transformation, where swift and decisive action can be made to address serious problems (Hay 1996). Thus, "crises" also generate opportunities—and in the case of this anthology—an opportunity to systematically think through the interacting social, material and political forces that impact traumatic brain injuries and sport.

The term "crises" also reflects debates over the multiple potential sources of brain injury risk in sports contexts, including but not limited to concussion. The term "concussion" is itself difficult to characterize as it has acquired immense cultural symbolism as an umbrella term for virtually all types of brain injury sustained in sport contexts. Indeed, public concern over diverse forms and outcomes of brain trauma, including concussive and sub-concussive hits, acute symptoms and long-term neurodegenerative disease, are frequently lumped together as part of sports' "concussion crisis." Despite its ubiquity across contemporary sports vernaculars, the precise meaning of the term "concussion" is still developing. Most formal definitions describe concussion as a type of brain injury induced by biomechanical forces resulting from a jolt or blow to the head or body. Common symptoms associated with concussion include headaches, dizziness, nausea, cognitive difficulties (e.g., memory loss or trouble concentrating), emotional disturbances, and sleep problems (McCrory, Meeuwisse et al. 2017).

Yet it is widely acknowledged that no "gold standard" criteria for concussion diagnosis currently exists. This is in part because the neurophysiological indicators of concussion are typically not visible through modern neuroimaging techniques and cannot be detected through even the most sophisticated biomedical tests. Instead, concussion diagnoses are made through systematic assessment of relevant symptoms and patients' self-reported observations (Harmon et al. 2019; Putukian 2011). There remains, therefore, considerable medical uncertainty across scientific definitions about whether "concussion" best describes a set of symptoms following brain trauma (cognitive difficulties, headache, dizziness etc.) or a specific type of structural damage to the brain—or some complex combination of both (McCrory, Meeuwisse et al. 2017; Romeu-Mejia et al. 2019; Satarasinghe et al. 2019; Mullally 2017; Gasquoine 2019). Scientists are hopeful that clarity around these issues will be provided through future developments in functional magnetic resonance imaging (fMRI) and other neuroimaging technologies, as well as improved testing methods in the areas of genetic and blood biomarkers (Putukian 2011; Romeu-Mejia et al. 2019).

The widespread use of the term "concussion" is further complicated by its corresponding classification as a "mild traumatic brain injury" (mTBI). The "mild" designation is meant to distinguish minor TBIs from "moderate" or "severe" injuries typically entailing prolonged loss of consciousness and substantial structural damage visible through neuroimaging (Malec et al. 2007). Concussion and mTBI are often used interchangeably in clinical and scientific settings, although scientists are engaged in debates about how and why these two terms coexist. Some researchers position concussion as a specific subset of mTBI with definitive neuropathological characteristics, whereas others have challenged the specificity of concussion as something neurologically or biomechanically distinct from any other type of mTBI. Overall, this ambiguity has generated substantial confusion and inconsistency across scientific studies and clinical guidelines (McCrory and Berkovic 2001; McCrory et al. 2013; Sharp and Jenkins 2015; Tator 2009; Gasquoine 2019; Harmon et al. 2013). Some commentators make strong arguments in favor of using mTBI instead of concussion, affirming that using the imprecise and colloquial term "concussion" risks understating the severity of brain injury and gives patients (and clinicians) false impressions that a swift recovery is inevitable (Sharp and Jenkins 2015; Comper et al. 2010; DeMatteo et al. 2010).

Interestingly, in the context of these debates, "concussion" remains the preferred terminology for describing brain injuries in sports settings. Use of the term "concussion" (rather than "TBI" or "mTBI") is almost universal among athletes, journalists and broadcasters, sports officials, and sports medicine practitioners. "Concussion," and "sport-related concussion" specifically, have also emerged as the preferred terms in many scientific studies about brain injuries sustained through sports participation. Although doctors and scientists have conducted formal research into the embodied effects of brain injury among athletes since at least the 1870s (Casper 2018a; Gasquoine 2019), the phrase "sport-related concussion" (SRC) came into widespread use among scientists in the early 2000s. The first PubMed citations for the term appear in 2000 and 2001, when a collection of mostly neurologists and neuropsychologists began publishing work describing sport-related concussion as a distinct scientific entity. Use of this language has risen immensely over the past two decades, reflected in the increase of PubMed citations from a meager 3 in 2001 to 110 in 2018 ("PubMed by Year: 'Sport-Related Concussion'" n.d.).

The prevalence of the "sport-related concussion" terminology developed alongside two important trends in the scientific study and clinical management of mTBI in sports. First, the founding of the subdiscipline of sports neuropsychology, a field almost exclusively dedicated to research and clinical practice concerning sport-related concussion (Echemendia and Julian 2001; Webbe 2010). Second, the 2001 establishment of a series of international conferences on sport-related concussion at which a select group of experts gather to produce "consensus statements" assessing the state of scientific evidence and outlining best practices for concussion management (e.g., McCrory, Meeuwisse, et al. 2017). The logic behind differentiating sport-related concussion from other forms of mTBI (such as those sustained in motor vehicle accidents or as injuries of war) was largely based on the view that sports collisions have distinct biomechanical characteristics, but also that athletes face unique pressures for returning to play (McCrory, Feddermann-Demont, et al. 2017).

The development of these research programs and scientific subdisciplines has thus responded to and informed calls for sport-specific management guidelines from sports organizations and governing bodies.

Together, these trends have cemented "sport-related concussion" as dominant terminology in studies of sports TBI. This language is indeed reflected in official position statements from high-profile groups such as the National Athletic Trainers Association in the United States and the American Medical Society for Sports Medicine (Guskiewicz et al. 2004; Harmon et al. 2019). Some researchers, however, have raised concerns that the scientific focus on "concussion" in sports medicine relies too heavily on treating identifiable, symptomatic injuries and ignores possible cumulative harm from asymptomatic, sub-concussive hits that may damage the brain over time (Tagge et al. 2018; Nauman and Talavage 2018). Yet, as Malcolm (2017) illustrates, the choice of terminology is also closely tied to the development of the international consensus statements on sport-related concussion, which have become widely influential in determining definitions and practices associated with sports TBI but are produced by a small group of experts at invite-only, "closed shop" meetings (See also McNamee, Partridge, and Anderson 2015). The term "sport-related concussion," then, operates as a form of scientific boundary-making, which separated sport as a distinct context for injury exposure, but also established a restrictive network of authoritative knowledge producers.

Although it is well beyond the scope of this introduction to thoroughly evaluate scientific justifications for these types of terminology choices, it is important to note that the constellation of terms used to describe brain injury in sports is contested and carries its own historical and epistemological complexities. Throughout this book, therefore, authors engage with terms and concepts based on the specific contexts and debates within which their work is situated. We, for example, use the dominant and recognizable term "concussion" in the title of this book and throughout the introduction to represent (and interrogate) the ubiquity of the concept in sports contexts; elsewhere in the collection, however, authors explore topics for which different terminology (TBI, sport-related concussion, CTE, etc.) best represents the scope and direction of their arguments. In sum, the analyses making up this book are not limited to "concussion" or "sport-related concussion" as defined in the contentious scientific literature on these topics; rather, they investigate the sociocultural implications of a broad spectrum of ways in which sport and brain injury are intertwined.

Forces of Impact: Contributions and Chapter Previews

Dominant definitions of concussion revolve around the impact of biomechanical forces on the tissues and neural circuitry of the brain. Yet this book investigates forces of a different kind: social, historical, economic, political, and ideological. While appearing external to the injury itself, these forces powerfully shape knowledge, experiences, and indeed the very materiality of brain injuries in sports. It is further important to note that the problem of concussion in sports has not only taken hold across media, politics, and public health domains, but scientific and cultural narratives about sports concussion profoundly influence conceptions of TBI beyond sport (Morrison and Casper 2016). As previously suggested and further evidenced in the above discussion of terminology, the issue of sport-related TBI is most frequently conceptualized through biomedical and scientific ways of knowing; chapters in this book interrogate the epistemological and ideological foundations of these knowledges, but also explore alternative ways of knowing and conceptualizing the complexity of concussion, often in conversation with biomedical and scientific paradigms. We have therefore divided *Sociocultural Examinations of Sports Concussions* into two sections, each examining distinct themes related to the critical study of sport-related brain injuries.

The initial section that follows, History, Health and Ethics, features four chapters, all of which center on the medical, political, epistemological, and moral stakes at play in debates about traumatic brain injuries in sports. Dominic Malcolm opens the section by investigating the medicalization of concussion and its possible link to Chronic Traumatic Encephalopathy (CTE), that is, probing the processes whereby everyday life, in this case regarding injured brains, are increasingly subject to medical attention and influence. Consequently, biomedical language comes to structure broader understandings of brain injuries while neurological protocols serve to identify and systematically treat sufferers. In "Concussion, Chronic Traumatic Encephalopathy, and the Medicalization of Sport," Malcolm explores the dynamics and consequences of this unstable process revealing the productive and limiting medical and ethical aspects of medicalization. On the one hand, amid resistance from sports organizations, such medicalization has helped to instill a sense of beneficence and a broader public awareness about sport-related brain trauma. On the other hand, such a biomedical focus tends to (re)standardize particular sets of practices and ways of knowing, which in turn limit alternatives while frequently suppressing individual differences and autonomy. This examination is additionally important in unveiling the hegemonic social practices involved in scientific renderings of TBI, a theme threaded throughout this collection.

The next three chapters use gridiron football as their site of investigation. This is not surprising given football's public and scholarly visibility, particularly within North American contexts, as well as recent concerns about the consequences of repeated, forceful collisions that help to constitute the sport. And yet, the next three chapters show that particular stakeholders including leagues, advertisers, players, parents, and an often-conciliatory media, frequently downplay or deny the embodied effects of concussions in an effort to maintain the sport's masculine status and associated lucrative markets. Kathleen Bachynski offers an historical analysis that sheds light upon contemporary legal, medical, and ethical trends related to the game. "'A Clear Conscience': Advertising Football Equipment and Responsibility for Injuries" traces twentieth century equipment manufacturers' marketing and legal campaigns promoting gridiron football and their products as sufficiently safe and culturally important. Their narratives did so through doublespeak: First by constructing equipment including helmets as crucial both to football and to the sport's apparent central role in instilling desired masculine values in boys. And yet, when faced with lawsuits, these same sporting goods manufacturers denied associations between their products and specific head injuries casting such injuries as matters of individual responsibility.

Fast-forwarding to contemporary times, we can see similar developments at work. In "Football Helmet Safety and the Veil of Standards" Daniel R. Morrison demonstrates how football helmet-rating bodies produce misleading information about helmet safety. While seemingly complete, the numerical values of the rating system are actually representative of the type of research conducted. In most cases, the rating tests measure the effect of linear forces on helmets. To date, research has not been conducted to capture the powerful impacts of rotational acceleration thought to better simulate the most damaging types of brain-jarring collisions which occur on the playing fields. Morrison thus unveils the limits of technological solutions, as well as the production of limited knowledge—even ignorance—which comprise these ratings. Grounded in a sociology of knowledge perspective, this analysis further implies that the "veil of standards" is complicit in numerically legitimating misinformation about helmets' ability to protect.

In "What Does the Precautionary Principle Demand of Us? Ethics, Population Health Policy, and Sports-Related TBI," Daniel Goldberg provides insights to more fully contextualize the critiques presented by Bachynski and Morrison. That is, actions by helmet manufacturers and associated rating bodies mobilize similar strategies used by those who are against the legislation seeking to curb youth football participation. Thus, each of these entities engage in the "manufacture of doubt" in following the lead of such industries as Big Tobacco in denying direct causal relationships between their products and ill health. In order to fight off potential state regulation and policy initiatives, opponents of attempts to curb youth football involvement activate uncertainty while suggesting that epidemiologic causation regarding football and TBI is the only evidence that matters. Since such causal inference is difficult to establish, Goldberg recommends applying the precautionary principle, a foundational concept within public health, to relax such standards of proof given the bodily harm that will ensue absent such an intervention.

In sum, analyses by Malcolm, Bachynski, Goldberg and Morrison collectively reveal that it is imperative to think through the claims created by individual and institutional actors given the ethical implications of such competing knowledge constructions. This is especially so given the personal, social, political, and economic costs and consequences of sport-related TBI.

The next section, the Politics of Trauma, Experience, and Research first documents the myriad of ways that concussion is experienced ranging from biographical disruptions to traumatic matters of life and death. The first three chapters of this section thus illustrate the diversity that constitutes

TBI experiences. The final two chapters hone in on the limitations of current research paradigms while calling for new interdisciplinary frameworks that better capture the complicated state of both experiences and the brain's materiality. In concert with analyses in the first section, these chapters tease out additional epistemological and political concerns.

In " 'I Kinda' Lost My Sense of Who I Was': Foregrounding Youths' Experiences in Critical Conversations about Sport-Related Concussions," authors William Bridel, Matt Ventresca, Danika Kelly, Kevin Viliunas, and Kathryn Schneider argue that first-person narratives produced by athletes must constitute a greater portion of research going forward. In that spirit, based upon qualitative interview materials, they explicate the narratives produced by athletes ages 10–14 at various stages of recovery from concussion. In particular, the athletes in their study frequently described important psychosocial effects or "biographical disruptions" including feelings of isolation, a loss of identity as an athlete, and worries about their future in sport. While pointing out sources of support, the authors connect these athletes' injury storylines to contradictory sport and health discourses around pain. Toward this end, the chapter helps to assert the ways in which sociocultural analyses of lived experiences are crucial components of "concussion knowledge," a reoccurring theme found throughout this section.

In "Trauma and Recovery: Violence Against Women in a 'Neurological Age'," Cathy van Ingen widens the scope of this anthology, applying a feminist lens to explore the experiences of sexual assault and violence survivors who participate in a non-contact, trauma-informed boxing program in Toronto, Ontario. Van Ingen's work also moves beyond medico-scientific concerns by also privileging the voices of women as an entry point to better understanding the complex lived experiences of trauma and survivorship. While non-contact boxing allows a way for survivors of intimate partner violence, including survivors of TBI, to reconnect with their minds and bodies, Van Ingen further argues the importance of moving beyond neurological understandings to challenge the patriarchal forces and actors which perpetuate trauma. Moreover, Van Ingen's scholarship exposes the bodily, political stakes involved in trauma and recovery as well as the absolute necessity of social change.

Sean Brayton and Michelle Helstein offer another ground-breaking examination of the often devastating, if not deadly, effects of trauma. In "The Athlete's Body and the Social Text of Suicide" Brayton and Helstein argue that the recent suicides involving professional football players and hockey enforcers are not simply personal choices of likely CTE sufferers to end their lives. Rather, these suicides are embodied social scripts that should be read as radical acts offering a "corporeal critique" which exposes professional sport as an economic enterprise built upon the use, abuse, and "disposability" of masculine athletic bodies as physical labor. In addition, this chapter points out the ongoing import of illuminating the economic and social forces that shape individual and institutional responses to brain injuries suffered in sports.

Two final chapters, the first by Kate Henne and the second by Matt Ventresca, conclude the anthology by exposing limitations of contemporary paradigms of sport-related TBI research. That is, both authors coherently and compellingly argue the need for alternative ontological and epistemological understandings of TBI beyond the dominance of biomedical models, which largely focus attention on men's collision sports. In "Brain Politics: Gendered Difference and Traumatic Brain Injury in Sport," Henne draws upon critical feminist frameworks to demonstrate how hegemonic understandings of sex and gender not only inform brain science but produce inadequate ways to address the messy symptoms and material consequences of sport-related TBI, especially regarding women's sports. Instead, she implores scholars to engage Feminist Science Studies to draw upon alternative frameworks that disrupt binary understandings of sex and injury while considering different ideologies and structures of opportunity that condition bodies differently. Thinking outside the gender binary will also help in theorizing the useful interventions currently sought by scientists, practitioners, and advocates for women's sports.

In "Beyond the Biopsychosocial: A Case for Critical Qualitative Concussion Research," Matt Ventresca also examines the incomplete scientific framing of concussion by dissecting the assumptions that undergird the biopsychosocial model of TBI. This analysis helps to expose the limitations of the compartmentalized, hegemonic "cause and effect" orientation of dominant TBI paradigms. Much as with other authors in this section, Ventresca additionally marshals the use of athletes' narratives as fodder for his interpretive qualitative investigation. In doing so, Ventresca unmasks the unruly character of brains and injuries beyond what can be reasonably captured within existing frameworks, which separate the biological from the psychological and the social forces impacting TBI. As an alternative, much as with Henne, Ventresca calls for fresh critical interdisciplinary insights, in this case, for prototypes better equipped to theorize the knotty co-construction of biological, psychological, and social aspects of injury.

Thanks to the deployment of socio-cultural insights, both Henne and Ventresca furthermore point toward the possibilities of more complicated understandings, not simply of TBI, but of the elastic materiality of embodied brains. Such an emphasis also disrupts western dualisms of nature-culture, mind-body, masculine-feminine, and biological-social. Much as with the critical neurological paradigm, these chapters reveal the essential plasticity of the brain, embodied and malleable, "itself a product of sociality, built through experiences and open to transformation" (Pitts-Taylor 2016, 2).

And finally, as co-editors we curated this anthology to explore and solidify the importance of sociocultural investigations in producing thorough understandings of concussion in sports. We were particularly committed to furthering critical conversations about the epistemological and ontological implications of traumatic brain injury. The authors in this volume confront crucial questions about what types of knowledge regarding concussion are counted as legitimate at the expense of others; who benefits from historical and contemporary ideas about the diagnosis and treatment of these injuries; and whose bodies and experiences are most valued in this context. Yet the chapters in this anthology also illustrate how brains *materialize* in concert with discourses and actions. The authors thus reveal the importance of onto-logical concerns in thinking through the *states of being* that emerge in and through brains and injuries. And yet, it is also important to emphasize that it is via critical consideration of knowledge and material realities that the com-mon ground between scientific, biomedical, and sociocultural disciplines emerge. A central aim of *Sociocultural Examinations of Sports Concussions* is to help deconstruct the traditional quantitative/qualitative or biological/psy-chosocial boundaries that typically define the study of concussion. Our hope is that this anthology encourages conversations which will promote sharing interdisciplinary knowledge, thus opening up new possibilities for collabo-ratively studying concussion and theorizing across multiple disciplines and forces of impact.

References

Anderson, Eric, and Edward M. Kian. 2012. "Examining Media Contestation of Masculinity and Head Trauma in the National Football League." *Men and Mas-culinities* 15 (2): 152–173.

Barad, Karen. 2007. *Meeting the Universe Halfway: Quantum Physics and the Entanglement of Matter and Meaning.* Raleigh, NC: Duke University Press.

Bell, Travis R., Janelle Applequist, and Christian Dotson-Pierson. 2019. *CTE, Media, and the NFL.* New York: Lexington Books.

Brayton, Sean, Michelle T Helstein, Mike Ramsey, and Nicholas Rickards. 2019. "Exploring the Missing Link Between the Concussion ' Crisis ' and Labor Poli-tics in Professional Sports." *Communication & Sport* 7 (1): 110–131.

Cantu, Robert, and Mark Hyman. 2012. *Concussions and Our Kids: America's Leading Expert on How to Protect Young Athletes and Keep Sports Safe.* New York: Mariner Books.

Carroll, Linda, and David Rosner. 2012. *The Concussion Crisis: Anatomy of a Silent Epidemic.* New York: Simon & Schuster.

Casper, Stephen T. 2018a. "Concussion : A History of Science and Medicine, 1870–2005." *Headache,* 58 (6): 795–810.

Casper, Stephen T. 2018b. "How the 1950s Changed Our Understanding of Traumatic Encephalopathy and Its Sequelae." *Canadian Medical Association Journal* 190 (5): E140 LP–E142 LP.

Cassilo, David, and Jimmy Sanderson. 2016. " 'I Don't Think It's Worth the Risk': Media Framing of the Chris Borland Retirement in Digital and Print Media." *Com-munication & Sport,* 1–25. https://doi.org/10.1177/2167479516654513.

Cassilo, David, and Jimmy Sanderson. 2018. "From Social Isolation to Becom-ing an Advocate: Exploring Athletes' Grief Discourse About Lived Concussion Experiences in Online Forums." *Communication & Sport,* July. https://doi.org/10.1177/2167479518790039.

Coakley, Jay. 2017. *Sports in Society: Issues and Controversies* (12th Ed.). New York: McGraw Hill.

Comper, Paul, Michael Hutchison, Sylvia Magrys, and Lynda Mainwaring. 2010. "Evaluating the Methodological Quality of Sports Neuropsychology Concussion Research : A Systematic Review." *Brain Injury* 24 (11): 1257–1271. https://doi.org/10.3109/02699052.2010.506854.

Dean, Nikolaus A. 2019. " 'Just Act Normal': Concussion and the (Re)Negotiation of Athletic Identity." *Sociology of Sport Journal* 36 (1): 22–31. https://doi.org/10.1123/ssj.2018-0033.

DeMatteo, Carol A., Steven E. Hanna, William J. Mahoney, Robert D. Hollenberg, Louise A. Scott, Mary C. Law, Anne Newman, Chia-Yu A. Lin, and Liqin Xu. 2010. "My Child Doesn't Have a Brain Injury, He Only Has a Concussion." *Pediatrics* 125 (2): 327 LP–334 LP. https://doi.org/10.1542/peds.2008-2720.

Diamond, Dan. 2014. "Obama Vs. Concussions: Why the White House Made Head Injuries a Presidential Issue." *Forbes*, May 29, 2014. www.forbes.com/sites/dandiamond/2014/05/29/obama-vs-concussions-why-the-white-house-made-head-injuries-a-presidential-issue/#6182e40a10ec.

Dumit, Joseph. 2004. *Picturing Personhood: Brain Scans and Biomedical Identity.* Princeton, NJ: Princeton University Press.

Echemendia, Ruben J, and Laura J Julian. 2001. "Mild Traumatic Brain Injury in Sports: Neuropsychology's Contribution to a Developing Field." *Neuropsychology Review* 11 (2): 69–88. https://doi.org/10.1023/A:1016651217141.

Fainaru-Wada, Mark, and Steve Fainaru. 2013. *League of Denial: The NFL, Concussions, and the Battle for Truth.* New York: Crown-Archetype.

Foucault, Michel. 1973. *The Birth of the Clinic.* New York: Routledge.

Furness, Zack. 2016. "Reframing Concussions, Masculinity, and NFL Mythology in League of Denial." *Popular Communication* 14 (1): 49–57.

Gasquoine, Philip Gerard. 2019. "Historical Perspectives on Evolving Operational Definitions of Concussive Brain Injury: From Railway Spine to Sport-Related Concussion." *The Clinical Neuropsychologist*, May, 1–18. https://doi.org/10.1080/13854046.2019.1621383.

Goldberg, Daniel S. 2012. "Mild Traumatic Brain Injury, the US National Football League, and the Manufacture of Doubt: An Ethical, Legal, and Historical Analysis." *Journal of Legal Medicine* 34 (2): 157–191.

Guarino, Ben. 2016. "Trump Knocks 'Softer' NFL Rules: Concussions—'Uh Oh, Got a Little Ding on the Head?' " *Washington Post*, October 13, 2016. www.washingtonpost.com/news/morning-mix/wp/2016/10/13/trump-just-criticized-the-nfls-softer-rules-intended-to-help-protect-players-from-traumatic-brain-injury/?utm_term=.c756391fd34d.

Guskiewicz, Kevin M., Scott L. Bruce, Robert C. Cantu, Michael S. Ferrara, James P. Kelly, Michael McCrea, Margot Putukian, and Tamara C Valovich McLeod. 2004. "National Athletic Trainers' Association Position Statement: Management of Sport-Related Concussion." *Journal of Athletic Training* 39 (3): 280–297. www.ncbi.nlm.nih.gov/pubmed/15514697.

Haraway, Donna. 1997. *Modest_Witness@Second_Millennium. FemaleMan ©_Meets_ OncoMouse™–Feminism and Technoscience.* New York: Routledge.

Hardes, Jennifer. 2017. "Governing Sporting Brains : Concussion, Neuroscience, and the Biopolitical Regulation of Sport Biopolitical Regulation of Sport." *Sport, Ethics and Philosophy* 11 (3): 1–13.

Harmon, Kimberly G., James R. Clugston, Katherine Dec, Brian Hainline, Stanley Herring, Shawn F Kane, Anthony P. Kontos, et al. 2019. "American Medical

Society for Sports Medicine Position Statement on Concussion in Sport." *British Journal of Sports Medicine* 53 (4): 213 LP–225 LP. https://doi.org/10.1136/bjsports-2018-100338.

Harmon, Kimberly G., Jonathan A. Drezner, Matthew Gammons, Kevin M Guskiewicz, Mark Halstead, Stanley A. Herring, Jeffrey S. Kutcher, Andrea Pana, Margot Putukian, and William O. Roberts. 2013. "American Medical Society for Sports Medicine Position Statement: Concussion in Sport." *British Journal of Sports Medicine* 47 (1): 15–26. https://doi.org/10.1136/bjsports-2012-091941.

Harrison, Emily. 2014. "The First Concussion Crisis: Head Injury and Evidence in Early American Football." *American Journal of Public Health* 104 (5): 822–833.

Hay, Colin. 1996. "Narrating Crisis: The Discursive Construction of the 'Winter of Discontent'." *Sociology* 30 (2): 253–277. https://doi.org/10.1177/00380 38596030002004.

Hull, Kevin, and Annelie Schmittel. 2014. "A Fumbled Opportunity? A Case Study of Twitter's Role in Concussion Awareness Opportunities During the Super Bowl." *Journal of Sport and Social Issues* 39 (1): 78–94.

Jasanoff, Sheila. 2005. *Designs on Nature: Science and Democracy in Europe and the United States*. Princeton: Princeton University Press. www.jstor.org/stable/j.ctt7spkz.

Kuhn, Andrew W., Aaron M. Yengo-Kahn, Zachary Y. Kerr, and Scott L. Zuckerman. 2017. "Sports Concussion Research, Chronic Traumatic Encephalopathy and the Media: Repairing the Disconnect." *British Journal of Sports Medicine* 51 (24): 1732 LP–1733 LP.

Liston, Katie, Mark McDowell, Dominic Malcolm, Andrea Scott-Bell, and Ivan Waddington. 2018. "On Being 'Head Strong': The Pain Zone and Concussion in Non-Elite Rugby Union." *International Review for the Sociology of Sport* 53 (6): 1012690216679966. https://doi.org/10.1177/1012690216679966.

Malcolm, Dominic. 2017. *Sport, Medicine, and Health: The Medicalization of Sport?* London: Routledge.

Malec, J.F., A.W. Brown, C.L. Leibson, J.T. Flaada, J.N. Mandrekar, N.N. Diehl, and P.K. Perkins. 2007. "The Mayo Classification System for Traumatic Brain Injury Severity." *Journal of Neurotrauma* 24 (9): 1417–1424.

McCrory, Paul R., and Samuel F. Berkovic. 2001. "Concussion." *Neurology* 57 (12): 2283 LP–2289 LP. https://doi.org/10.1212/WNL.57.12.2283.

McCrory, Paul R., Nina Feddermann-Demont, Jiří Dvořák, J. David Cassidy, Andrew McIntosh, Pieter E. Vos, Ruben J. Echemendia, Willem Meeuwisse, and Alexander A. Tarnutzer. 2017. "What Is the Definition of Sports-Related Concussion: A Systematic Review." *British Journal of Sports Medicine* 51 (11): 877 LP–887 LP. https://doi.org/10.1136/bjsports-2016-097393.

McCrory, Paul R., Willem H. Meeuwisse, Ruben J. Echemendia, Grant L. Iverson, Jiří Dvořák, and Jeffrey S. Kutcher. 2013. "What Is the Lowest Threshold to Make a Diagnosis of Concussion?" *British Journal of Sports Medicine* 47 (5): 268 LP–271 LP. https://doi.org/10.1136/bjsports-2013-092247.

McCrory, Paul R., Willem H. Meeuwisse, Jiří Dvorak, Mark Aubry, Julian Bailes, Steven Broglio, Robert C. Cantu, et al. 2017. "Consensus Statement on Concussion in Sport—the 5 Th International Conference on Concussion in Sport Held in Berlin, October 2016." *British Journal of Sports Medicine* 51 (11): 1–10.

McDonald, Mary G., and Susan Birrell. 1999. "Reading Sport Critically: A Methodology for Interrogating Power." *Sociology of Sport Journal* 16 (4): 283–300.

McGannon, Kerry R., Sarah M. Cunningham, and Robert J. Schinke. 2013. "Understanding Concussion in Socio-Cultural Context: A Media Analysis of a National Hockey League Star's Concussion." *Psychology of Sport and Exercise* 14: 891–899.

McNamee, Michael J., Bradley Partridge, and Lynley Anderson. 2015. "Concussion in Sport: Conceptual and Ethical Issues." *Kinesiology Review* 4 (2): 190–202. https://doi.org/10.1123/kr.2015-0011.

Mills, C. Wright. 1959. *The Sociological Imagination*. New York: Oxford University Press.

Morrison, Daniel R., and Monica J. Casper. 2016. "Gender, Violence, and Brain Injury in and Out of the NFL: What Counts as Harm?" In *Football, Culture, and Power*, edited by David Leonard, Kimberly B. George, and Wade Davis, 156–175. New York: Routledge.

Mullally, William J. 2017. "Concussion." *The American Journal of Medicine* 130 (8): 885–892. https://doi.org/10.1016/j.amjmed.2017.04.016.

Nauman, Eric A., and Thomas M. Talavage. 2018. "Chapter 24 — Subconcussive Trauma." In *Sports Neurology*, edited by Brian Hainline, and Robert ABT—Handbook of Clinical Neurology Stern, 158:245–255. Elsevier. https://doi.org/https://doi.org/10.1016/B978-0-444-63954-7.00024-0.

Oates, Thomas P. 2017. *Football and Manliness: An Unauthorized Feminist Account of the NFL*. Chicago, IL: University of Illinois Press.

Pitts-Taylor, Victoria. 2016. *The Brain's Body: Neuroscience and Corporeal Politics*. Durham, NC: Duke University Press.

"PubMed by Year: 'Sport-Related Concussion.'" n.d. *PubMed by Year*, June 28, 2019. https://esperr.github.io/pubmed-by-year/?q1=%22Sport-related concussion%22&endyear=2018.

Putukian, Margot. 2011. "The Acute Symptoms of Sport-Related Concussion: Diagnosis and On-Field Management." *Clinics in Sports Medicine* 30 (1): 49–61. https://doi.org/10.1016/j.csm.2010.09.005.

Rebecca D., Boneau, Brian K. Richardson, and Joseph McGlynn. 2018. "'We Are a Football Family': Making Sense of Parents' Decisions to Allow Their Children to Play Tackle Football." *Communication & Sport*, December. https://doi.org/10.1177/2167479518816104.

Reed, Ken. 2017. "Promising News on the Concussion Front." *Huffington Post*, March 2, 2017. www.huffpost.com/entry/promising-news-on-the-con_b_9361268.

Roderick, Martin. 1998. "The Sociology of Risk, Pain and Injury: A Comment on the Work of Howard L. Nixon II." *Sociology of Sport Journal* 15 (1): 64–79.

Roderick, Martin. 2006. "The Sociology of Pain and Injury in Sport: Main Perspectives and Problems." In *Pain and Injury in Sport*, edited by Sigmund Loland, Berit Skirstad, and Ivan Waddington, 17–35. New York: Routledge.

Romeu-Mejia, Rafael, Christopher C. Giza, and Joshua T. Goldman. 2019. "Concussion Pathophysiology and Injury Biomechanics." *Current Reviews in Musculoskeletal Medicine* 12 (2): 105–116. https://doi.org/10.1007/s12178-019-09536-8.

Rose, Nikolas, and Joelle M. Abi-Rached. 2013. *Neuro: The New Brain Sciences and the Management of the Mind*. Princeton, NJ: Princeton University Press.

Safai, Parissa. 2003. "Healing the Body in the 'Culture of Risk': Examining the Negotiation of Treatment Between Sport Medicine Clinicians and Injured Athletes in Canadian Intercollegiate Sport." *Sociology of Sport Journal* 20 (2): 127–146.

Satarasinghe, Praveen, D. Kojo Hamilton, Robert J. Buchanan, and Michael T. Koltz. 2019. "Unifying Pathophysiological Explanations for Sports-Related Concussion and Concussion Protocol Management: Literature Review." *Journal of Experimental Neuroscience* 13, January: 1179069518824125. https://doi.org/10.1177/1179069518824125.

Sharp, David J., and Peter O. Jenkins. 2015. "Concussion Is Confusing Us All." *Practical Neurology* 15 (3): 172 LP–186 LP. http://pn.bmj.com/content/15/3/172.abstract.

Stewart, William, Kieren Allinson, Safa Al-Sarraj, Corbin Bachmeier, Karen Barlow, Antonio Belli, Mark P. Burns, et al. 2019. "Primum Non Nocere: A Call for Balance When Reporting on CTE." *The Lancet Neurology* 18 (3): 231–233. https://doi.org/10.1016/S1474-4422(19)30020-1.

Tagge, Chad A., Andrew M. Fisher, Olga V. Minaeva, Amanda Gaudreau-, Juliet A. Moncaster, Xiao-lei Zhang, Mark W. Wojnarowicz, et al. 2018. "Concussion, Microvascular Injury, and Early Tauopathy in Young Athletes After Impact Head Injury and an Impact Concussion Mouse Model." *Brain* 141, February: 422–458.

Tator, Charles H. 2009. "Let's Standardize the Definition of Concussion and Get Reliable Incidence Data." *Canadian Journal of Neurological Sciences/Journal Canadien Des Sciences Neurologiques* 36 (4): 405–406. https://doi.org/doi:10.1017/S031716710000771X.

Theberge, Nancy. 2008. " 'Just a Normal Bad Part of What I Do': Elite Athletes' Accounts of the Relationship Between Health and Sport." *Sociology of Sport Journal* 25: 206–222.

Ventresca, Matt. 2019. "The Curious Case of CTE: Mediating Materialities of Traumatic Brain Injury." *Communication & Sport* 7 (2): 135–156. https://doi.org/10.1177/2167479518761636.

Ventresca, Matt. 2020. "The Tangled Multiplicities of CTE: Scientific Uncertainty and the Infrastructures of Traumatic Brain Injury." In *Sports, Society, and Technology: Bodies, Practices, and Knowledge Production*, edited by Jennifer Sterling, and Mary G. McDonald. New York: Palgrave Macmillan.

Webbe, Frank M. 2010. "Introduction to Sport Neuropsychology." In *The Handbook of Sport Neuropsychology*, edited by Frank M. Webbe, 1–16. New York: Springer Publishing Company.

Young, Kevin. 2004. "Sports-Related Pain and Injury: Sociological Notes." In *Sporting Bodies, Damaged Selves: Sociological Studies of Sports-Related Injury*, edited by Kevin Young, 1–25. Oxford, UK: Elsevier.

Part II

History, Health, Ethics

2 Concussion, Chronic Traumatic Encephalopathy, and the Medicalization of Sport

Dominic Malcolm

Sports participants have experienced head injuries of various types since sports participation began. Throughout the early history of sport are numerous references like the description of the "Brompton Gents" who "retired home with broken heads and black eyes" following a cricket match in England in 1731 (cited in Malcolm 2013). But due to the nature of the then contemporary medical understanding of head injury, such concerns were largely expressed in relation to the release of blood from the head. Other signs of brain injury—like amnesia, disorientation, or loss of consciousness—because they were/are usually transitory and resolve spontaneously, were not believed by doctors to be particularly significant. And it is as a consequence of later modes of medical understanding that firstly concussion, and latterly its potential link with Chronic Traumatic Encephalopathy (CTE), have risen to the fore. It is in light of the temporal specificity of medical understandings of concussion that any sociocultural examination of this phenomenon must be grounded. Generating such an analytical framework is the fundamental aim of this chapter.

Some excellent work in this regard has already been started (Bachynski 2019; Shurley and Todd 2012). Emily Harrison's (2014) analysis of "the first concussion crisis" shows how doctors treating American college football players around the turn of the twentieth century began to chart both the frequency of concussion and the potential for long-term behavioural consequences. Harvard team doctors recorded an incidence of almost one concussion per game among football players during the 1906 season. The impact of such concerns was inhibited by the (continued) absence of visual evidence of brain damage and lack of empirical evidence of a link between concussion and the subsequent "insanity" and "alcoholism" that some scientists claimed it entailed. However, ultimately, the crisis was averted through the mobilization of economic interests, as colleges began to see sport as an important recruitment tool and attempts were made to emphasize the capacity of football to develop important masculine qualities. Some evidence of the scale of harm was hidden from public view, while technical "solutions" such as enhanced protective equipment and improved playing technique meant that the weaknesses of the body of biomedical evidence could be exploited and the issue dismissed.

Others have rightly pointed to the more sustained and, to some extent, successful campaigns against boxing. The health hazards of boxing first became subject to explicit and formalized medical concern in 1893. In this year, *The Lancet* (a leading UK medical journal), drew readers' attention to the death of three boxers, all of whom had experienced head injuries of some form (Sheard 1998). The key medical development, however, occurred in 1928 when pathologist Harrison Martland introduced the term "punch drunk" to describe former boxers who exhibited symptoms of neurological deficit. Martland could only speculate about the underlying neurological damage, but the medical community's adoption of the term *dementia pugilistica* in 1937 shows that his ideas nevertheless gained widespread acceptance (Castellani and Perry 2017). Indeed, Weinberg and Arond (1952), in one of the founding studies in the sociocultural analysis of sport, described the prevalence of long-term neurological damage as a salient feature of the "occupational subculture of boxing." In the United Kingdom, the 1969 "Roberts Report" not only concluded that there were approximately 200 severely "punch drunk" boxers across the UK, but correlated incidence with career length and fight exposure. Given how long and widely these ideas have been accepted, and their degree of "seriousness," it is remarkable that until recently sociologists have paid little attention to the lived experience of brain injury amongst current and former sports participants.

In what follows I present a developmental (as opposed to historical) account of the changing place and role of concussion in sport. A developmental approach focuses on the study of social processes and thus should be seen as distinct from a historical approach which may, for instance, seek to identify a range of particular instances that have occurred over time (Malcolm 2015). The framework I deploy to structure an understanding of concussion, and the central process interrogated, is that of *medicalization*. First, I explore the notion of medicalization, identifying the three distinct domains or levels at which researchers have identified evidence of this process (the conceptual, institutional and interactional levels), and outlining how the concept has previously been applied to the study of sport. Subsequently, I look at the way in which different dimensions of medicalization are evident in the development of concussion and CTE as major public issues in sport. Specifically, I argue that the multi-layered processes of medicalization are often uneven and sometimes competing and contradictory. As we will see, the particular concerns generated by emergent findings in relation to CTE (the pathology of which is currently poorly defined) have created a demand for action that is specific and empirically measurable and, thus, must be delivered through the policing of concussion at the institutional and interactional levels (at the levels of policy and through people respectively). This mismatch or incongruence between different domains of medicalization serves to fuel social concerns about brain injuries in sport. The conclusion reflects upon the consequences of the medicalization of concussion and CTE, particularly in relation to medical ethical principles.

Medicalization

Medicalization can be defined as the process whereby "more and more of everyday life has come under medical domain, influence and supervision" (Zola 1983, 295). Initially a discourse about medicalization arose in relation to the growing role of medicine in defining and treating certain 'deviant' practices. Deviance, sociologically speaking, is a behaviour that violates social norms, and it was on this basis, for instance, that Talcott Parsons (1975) conceptualized illness as a form of deviance; that is to say, when someone is socially recognized as being ill, expectations about 'normal' behaviour are suspended (e.g., the ill are excused from working). Latterly, however, medicalization has been evoked to describe how a range of natural aspects of the life-course (e.g., childbirth and ageing) have moved from the lay sphere of expertise into the domain of medical practice. Thus, sports medicine as a discrete area of practice, could be described as one manifestation of medicalization; historically, medical specialists have replaced the athletes and trainers/coaches previously responsible for the treatment of conditions incurred through, or limiting participation in, sport (Waddington 1996). The central role that clinicians are now required to play in making decisions about the "fitness" of those incurring brain injuries to play on is an example of the "policing" of deviance that medicine is called upon to exercise in the realm of sport. Players with medically diagnosed injuries are not expected to continue playing, and those with brain injuries are positively restricted in their attempts to do so.

Medicalization "cannot and should not be read as questioning the value of medicine" (Williams et al. 2018, 775), but it can and should focus on both the process and consequences of a phenomenon becoming defined as a medical problem (Conrad 2015). Thus, fundamental questions might include the consequences of using medicine as a tool of social control or medical professional expansion. Illich (1975), for instance, argued that medicalization meant that the profession not only cured illness and relieved suffering but created iatrogenesis; that is, medically caused (or exacerbated) illness and/or social problems. Sheard's (2003) argument that the introduction of head guards in boxing may have successfully reduced cuts to the head but unintentionally increased the incidence of brain injury is a pertinent example of iatrogenesis. But the depiction of medicalization as intentional and imperialistic which characterized early sociological accounts floundered as it became clear that the ability and ambition of members of the medical profession to expand their social influence was easily exaggerated. For instance, De Swaan (1989) introduced the term "reluctant imperialism" to capture the recognition within the medical profession that being called on to adjudicate on social conflicts (e.g., fitness to play sport) created sometimes unnecessary or somewhat "peripheral" problems for the profession and threatened to undermine the sense of collectivism which has historically contributed to medicine's social power. Indicatively, Malcolm (2009) cites clinicians who seriously damaged previously good relationships with key players through the diagnosis of concussion, thereby weakening their status and occupational security within what is already a notably precarious position (Malcolm 2006).

Conrad has more recently suggested that while the broader medicalization process continues to develop (if not extends in terms of reach and speed with which "issues" are medicalized), emphasis has shifted as the "engines of medicalization" proliferate and doctors move from drivers to "gatekeepers" of the process (Conrad 2007, 142). Consequently, medicalization has come to be understood as potentially evident on three different levels: conceptual, institutional and interactional (Conrad 1992). Respectively, these are evident when: medical vocabularies come to structure public understanding of particular aspects of social life; medical practices are used to administer social problems; and medical actors become central to the "cure" of social problems (Halfmann 2011). Any analysis of the different levels of medicalization, or the cultural domains in which such processes are manifest, should also recognize the relative willingness of "patient" groups to embrace or resist medicalization. Considered in this multidimensional way, medicalization can be: partial or extensive; the intended or unintended outcome of human action; and/or occur either with or without the medical profession. Different branches of medicine are uniquely equipped to *achieve* medicalization, and potentially differentially oriented in their aspirations to *seek* medicalization.

It is important, therefore, to see medicalization as a process that has both *enabling* and *constraining* effects. The absence of medicalization—where medical recognition is withheld, research funding is limited, treatments are underdeveloped, and public sympathies are muted—can be equally if not more incapacitating and distressing for those involved. The frustrations experienced by Mike Webster (the former National Football League player and the first person diagnosed with CTE), as he and his family sought compensation for his declining cognitive state, are a case in point (Fainaru-Wada and Fainaru 2013). Similarly, it is important to avoid the representation of medicine as a monolith. The sub-specialty of sports medicine holds an ambiguous position in relation to the broader profession. Not only has its status been weakened by its historic commitment to multidisciplinarity and limited by only somewhat partial state support in many Western nations (Malcolm 2017), but it is also necessarily linked to the division of medicine into specialisms and thus subject to intra-professional as well as interprofessional conflicts (Malcolm and Scott 2011). Specifically in relation to concussion and CTE, for instance, there are elements of friction between the sports medicine community and that of neurology and neuroscience (see, e.g., Sharp and Jenkins' (2015) call for the largely sport-related term "concussion," to be withdrawn from clinical use and replaced with a single classification system for traumatic brain injury (TBI)). Thirdly, it is important to recognize the social reforms that have developed out of sociological critiques of medicalization, ranging from the proletarianization of medicine (changing work conditions, de-skilling through an extended division of labour) to de-professionalization (greater degrees of administrative control, jurisdictional contestation by members of other healthcare professions, as evidenced by the burgeoning market for books providing complementary and alternative medical treatments for concussion). Finally, it is essential to see the degree of interdependence that is fundamental to the medicine-sport relationship. Sports medicine, as both an area of scientific scholarship and a community of practitioners, is highly dependent on the sports community for both its existence and validation. More recent moves towards the public health potential of exercise have served to expand sports medicine's social influence through a broader public health remit, but it remains the case that without the access to special populations that "sport" can grant, and the social status derived from working with an extremely high-profile group of celebrities, sports medicine would have a much more limited aura of expertise.

The Medicalization of Sport

The application of medicalization to sport first emerged in Waddington and Murphy's (1992) analysis of the development of the use of performance-enhancing drugs. As one of the first attempts to understand "doping" in relation to the "supply" of medical assistance (rather than simply athlete demand), it drew on a conceptualization of medicalization as the expanding realm of medical influence (although equally a case could have been made here for medicalization in the sense of the requirement of medicine to take a central role in the policing of this "deviant" behaviour). The publication of this text coincided with that of John Hoberman's seminal developmental account of sports medicine, *Mortal Engines* (1992), and the two theses are highly compatible. Hoberman (1992, 19) for instance, notes that "sport and medicine . . . developed a symbiotic relationship during the twentieth century," first with athletes being used as extreme or atypical cases that revealed the limits of human physical potential, and latterly with medical experimentation advancing the performance-orientation of elite sport. Waddington's (1996) subsequent analysis of the development of sports medicine literature illustrates how, in line with this process, athletes came to be defined as a distinct population whose need for continuous medical support is akin to the needs of the chronically ill; in other words, the widespread acceptance of the idea that "athletes require routine medical supervision, not because they necessarily have a clearly defined pathology but . . . simply because they are athletes" (Waddington 1996, 197). Latterly Beamish and Ritchie (2006, 8) extended the reach of this argument, suggesting that the rational pursuit of enhanced human athletic performance (and the quest for commercially rewarded and/or nationally prestigious victory), has led sport to become "an intensive, exhaustive occupation where athletes are fully embroiled in sophisticated training regimes utilizing scientifically developed technologies that create long-term physiological and personality changes as they progress through the high-stakes, "winner-takes-all" road to the pinnacle of world-class sport." For Beamish and Ritchie, therefore, medicalization is not simply a discrete element of the development of sport, but a fundamental driving force of its contemporary development.

Other examples of the medicalization of sport include the (mandatory) health screening programmes operant in certain (mainly European) nations, the introduction and development of various forms of participant sex-testing, and the systems of disability classification which underpin the very existence of Paralympic sport. *Sport, Medicine and Health: the medicalization of sport?* (Malcolm 2017), provides the most extensive interrogation of the relationship between sport and medicalization produced to date. Following a broad review of the interdependence of sport, medicine and health, embracing the organizational development of sports (and exercise) medicine, the provision and practice of elite sports medicine, the role of exercise in public health campaigns, the response of target populations to such campaigns, and the specific issues relating to concussion and cardiac screening, the book concludes that:

> The sum of these processes is that the medicalization of sport is far more apparent (or at least extensive) at the conceptual level than it is in relation to the actual practice of medical techniques and/or the engagement of patients. . . . Constraining the more holistic medicalization of sport has been the triad of sport's relative autonomy, intra-medical conflicts which have retarded the development and restricted the jurisdictional domain of sports medicine and state concerns to harness escalating healthcare costs. Medicine has, therefore, been more central to defining aspects of sport using its own nomenclature and paradigmatic assumptions than it has been in public intervention and implementation.
>
> (Malcolm 2017, 168–169)

Public debates regarding concussion have exponentially grown since this work was published. Significant here is the connection between concussion and CTE, which began, as noted above, in relation to boxing and American football, but which now engulfs a range of contact and collision sports and all the other major football codes: namely association (or soccer), rugby (union and league) and Australian Rules football. What many now perceive as a crisis in sport has spread not only in geographical terms but also in terms of both potential causes *and* consequences. Which particular aspects of these activities— from high-force, head-on collisions, to the relatively minor (but potentially frequent) impacts incurred when heading a 430-gram soccer ball—lead to which particular consequences—from short-lived and temporary forms of neurocognitive disruption to longer term, life-changing conditions such as dementia or amyotrophic lateral sclerosis (ALS)—remains to be fully established. For instance, in a recent letter published in *Lancet Neurology*, Stewart et al. (2019, 231) call for "balance" in media reporting on CTE and note that "CTE has yet to be fully defined. . . [the] diagnostic criteria are no more than preliminary. We have an incomplete understanding of the extent or distribution of pathology." Fundamentally though, the potential for activities which have historically been assumed to be "healthy" to lead to dementia—described as "one of the global health priorities of our age" (Hillman and Latimer 2017, 1)—has only increased the relevance of an analysis based on the concept of medicalization. Indeed, what makes these conditions stand out as examples or exemplars of this process is the degree to which they resonate with each level of the broader social process of the medicalization of sport. To illustrate this, the next section explores how the medicalization of concussion and CTE is evident at the conceptual, institutional, and interactional levels of analysis.

The Medicalization of Concussion and CTE

Conceptual Level

The conceptual level of medicalization is evident when medical vocabularies come to structure public understandings of a phenomenon. Because modern societies are so heavily influenced by media representations, the latter inevitably play a very significant part in the dissemination of medical ideas to lay audiences. Thus, analyses of the portrayal of some of the higher-profile cases of concussion have highlighted the role of media in disseminating certain messages about concussion. McGannon et al. (2013), for instance, explored the representation of the National Hockey League's Sidney Crosby and his return to play following multiple concussions in 2011. They argue that a somewhat "limited" understanding of concussion emerged (in relation to the depiction of the condition as an essentially physical injury with physiological rather than psychological effects), but equally that the public were exposed to media messages about both the limitations of existing biomedical understanding and the potential seriousness of concussion. Combined, these created the necessity to raise awareness among the public, and journalists took this opportunity to open a wider political debate about whether sports organizations were doing enough to address the issue. In defining Crosby's rehabilitation in terms of neurological monitoring of physiological symptoms, media representations fundamentally positioned concussion within medical terms rather than the psychological, social, and cultural domains that provide a more holistic perspective to what remains a relatively poorly understood condition (McGannon et al. 2013).

The degree to which medical notions come to structure public understanding is, however, more directly evident in the content of social media due to the more democratic authorship of content. Several studies have, for instance, identified how Twitter has become a significant medium for concussion-related content, with major themes being users' tweets about their own personal experiences of brain injury, news about incidence among professional athletes, dissemination of medical research, and debates about policy and injury prevention (Workewych et al. 2017). The growth in the quantity of concussion-related social media content can be seen by comparing the surveys of Sullivan et al. (2012) who identified 3,488 tweets in 7 days in July 2010, with Workewych et al. (2017), who discovered nearly 300,000 tweets within a month (9 June–9 July) just three years later (though notably both studies took place in the off-season for the NHL, NFL, and northern hemisphere rugby union, which have, perhaps, had the highest profile concussion incidents). While the vast majority of tweets (83%) use medical rather than colloquial descriptors (Workewych 2017), a number of researchers have expressed concern about the accuracy of the content disseminated (Ahmed et al. 2017; Kuhn et al. 2017; Workewych et al. 2017).

Such concerns are to some extent predicated on a misplaced degree of faith in the certainty of medical knowledge about these conditions. Indeed, media surveys conducted by biomedically oriented researchers complain of both the media's tendency to downplay the seriousness of concussion (e.g., the use of modifying terms such as "blow to the head" to project potentially "softer" implications of the injury, Ahmed and Hall 2017) and media's "propogat[ion of] an agenda of one-sided headline news and a sensationalised state of fear" (Kuhn et al. 2017, 1732). But reporting inaccuracies and sensationalism are intertwined as evidenced by the somewhat contradictory outcomes of athlete resistance to concussion-related public health campaigns (see discussion of medicalization at the interactional level) and the public self-diagnoses of CTE amongst former elite athletes (Ventresca 2019). While Caron et al. (2013) note that there is a considerable degree of overlap between the documented symptoms of post-concussion syndrome and the experience of retirement (depression, anxiety, isolation, and even suicidal ideation), a similar parallel could be drawn between responses to retirement and the behavioral, cognitive, and emotional manifestations which media reports have implicitly or explicitly linked to the contraction of CTE. These instances are indicative of the potential iatrogenic effects of medicalization. Limited and uncertain medical knowledge creates a framework through which relatively routine aspects of the life course (i.e., retirement) can be (mis)interpreted as the initial symptoms of not only a longer-term chronic illness, but one of the most feared conditions of our age.

Despite the ambiguities and inconsistencies evident across media reports, and the ultimate privileging of scientific understandings within these accounts (Ventresca 2019), media representations are key markers of medicalization at the conceptual level. Media are particularly keen to focus on technological "solutions" for concussion, such as the development of wearable impact-measuring equipment, virtual reality concussion assessment tools, and the illusive search for a biomarker of concussion (Wilson 2019). What these developments have in common is an underpinning assumption that concussion will, eventually, be knowable and understandable as a specific corporeal condition amenable to medical control. They are premised on the belief that the more precise understanding of the effects of external forces on the brain or a reliable diagnostic tool are potential outcomes. Yet history shows us that biomedicine is a field in which uncertainty is endemic (Fox 2000). Indeed, advances in the medical understanding of concussion have been notably slow in recent decades and many of the changes made to concussion consensus statements are more the product of social concerns than shifting empirical evidence (Malcolm 2020; see next section).

In order to comprehend public understandings of concussion and CTE then, it is important to locate media discourses within the "neuroscientific turn in contemporary biomedicine" (Ventresca 2019, 4). Developments in neuroscience are perceived as having the potential to unlock the final frontier of medical understanding. They rely on representing the functioning of the brain in particular ways and, while CTE is by no means at the forefront of these processes, being both *un*amenable to modern imaging techniques and only diagnosable post-mortem, the prominence of the Boston University "brain bank" studies in the public imagination is clear evidence of the foregrounding of biomedicine. The caution which even this group of researchers uses when discussing their research findings (specifically in acknowledging the absence of proof relating to a causal link between CTE and any specific activity or outcome, e.g. Mez et al. 2017), is often disregarded in the simplified accounts disseminated to and by the public on social media. Consequently, the key "causal link" question both exaggerates the power of (contemporary) science to explain all aspects of the human condition and allows the defenders of sporting practices to defer implementing radical changes until such "proof" is available. Indicative of the power of this conceptual level of medicalization has been the successful legal action brought forth by NFL players in 2012, for although the case was settled in the absence of compelling evidence of a sport-concussion-CTE link, an explicit assumption underlying the settlement was that it was merely a matter of time before neuroscience would produce such compelling evidence (Hardes 2017).

Institutional Level

Institutional level medicalization is evident where medical practices are used to "manage" corporeal conditions. The initial moves towards the medical management of concussion were, however, highly problematic. For instance, in the late 1990s some scientists argued that existing research on concussion in sport was "anecdotal . . . bizarre rather than reflecting established medical principles" and that the field was plagued by a "neuromythology" derived from folk wisdom, methodologically flawed medical research, and media exposés of athletes' experiences of head trauma and/or brain injury (McCrory 2001, 82). It was further noted how the disjointed development of the field of concussion research had become counterproductive to effective medical management. Specifically, the design and publication of an extensive range of severity scales for assessing the condition provided contradictory advice about whether concussion injuries should be graded according to the presence/absence of particular symptoms (rather than their duration) and led to confusion among clinicians about which advice to follow when managing the condition (McCrory 1999).

At the beginning of the twenty-first century, however, a process began whereby the science of concussion would become more unified and thus coherent. The single most tangible marker of this development was the establishment in 2001 of a series of international conferences on sports concussion which have since produced a succession of Agreement/Consensus Statements on Concussion in Sport. Initially organized under the auspices of the International Ice Hockey Federation (IIHF), the Federation Internationale de Football Associations (FIFA), and the International Olympic Committee, these consensus statements have facilitated a degree of regulatory convergence across sports. The production of Concussion in Sport Guidelines (CISG) has led to a standardized definition of concussion, which, significantly, concludes that a direct blow to the head and loss of consciousness (LOC) should *not* be deemed diagnostic prerequisites of concussion (indeed it is frequently cited that approximately only 10% of concussions entail LOC, e.g. Broglio et al. 2010). The protocol produced by the CISG has been adopted by most international sports governing bodies and has therefore become the global "gold standard" for concussion management. It recommends that athletes: undergo baseline cognitive testing; have concussion symptoms assessed using a standardized Sports Concussion Assessment Tools (SCAT, now in its fourth iteration and more detailed and extensive than ever); and be wholly asymptomatic throughout a six-phase graduated RTP programme, lasting a minimum of six days and overseen by a medical practitioner. A fundamental logic of these protocols, therefore, is that while there is a need to protect individuals from incurring further damage when concussed (i.e., second impact syndrome), it is less crucial to protect individuals from incurring multiple concussions over an extended period of time (i.e., CTE).

In light of the prior discussion of the contentious evidential basis for CTE (and how this enables resistance to calls for the implementation of radical changes in sport), it is interesting to note that there is relatively little empirical evidence to substantiate the effectiveness of concussion protocols now in place. Criticisms have been voiced, for instance in relation to: diagnostic inclusion criteria that are too broad and therefore likely to capture multiple other conditions; the lack of supportive evidence for prescribing physical and cognitive rest; and a flawed graduated RTP protocol that is not operational because most people are never fully asymptomatic of the inclusion criteria (Craton and Leslie 2014, 93). Even the authoritative consensus statements have noted that the "science of concussion is evolving" (McCrory et al. 2013, 250) and the consensus statements are replete with provisos and reservations stressing how many areas of concussion science contain uncertainties.

But such flaws and evidential weaknesses have not stopped the widespread adoption of these protocols across the sports community, albeit with some sport-specific modifications. For instance, in 2011 the Australian Football League (AFL) and National Rugby League (NRL) implemented concussion management systems based on the CISG. To encourage conservative management, rugby league teams were awarded an additional substitution for when a player is withdrawn exhibiting concussion symptoms. Rugby union has, too, adopted the CISG but supplements this protocol with the more contentious "head injury bin," which permits temporary substitutions to create extra time for the diagnosis of concussion. Ironically, given FIFA's early involvement in the process, the adoption of the CISG in football/soccer has been relatively slow. For instance, the English Football Association only adopted use of the SCAT and the six-phase graduated RTP (although not time-limited) in its 2012–13 regulations, and it was not until a number of high-profile incidents (particularly involving the Tottenham Hotspur goalkeeper Hugo Lloris, who completed a match after having clearly been knocked unconscious for a significant period), that the regulations were revised to mirror the "gold standard" protocol noted above. It is testimony to the power and authority of the medical profession, and indicative of how socially pervasive the medicalization process is, that these protocols, based on little more than the ethical principle of "first do no harm," are so widely adopted.

Perhaps the clearest indication of the medicalization of concussion at the institutional level, however, is the licence and mandate granted to these medical practices through state legislature. At the forefront of this development has been the Lystedt Law, which, since its introduction in Washington State in 2009, has been adopted across the United States. While there is considerable cross-state diversity in the specific terms of this legislation, implemented measures include concussion training/education of coaches, players, and parents, the compulsory notification of parents when a concussion is suspected or diagnosed, and a requirement that players must be cleared by a licensed physician or someone trained in brain injury management before returning to play. Proposals to introduce parallel nationwide legislation in Canada (as an extension of the province of Ontario's 2018 Rowan's Law) illustrate this as an ongoing process.

Interactional Level

Interactional levels of medicalization are evident when medical actors become centrally placed as the ultimate "cure" of the social problem of concussion. Indicatively, the various SCAT tools are premised on the identification of physicians as the appropriate professionals to take responsibility for concussion management (a role augmented by the increasing complexity of the SCAT). Most fundamentally, perhaps, the primacy of medicine is established by the continued provision in the CISG of all RTP decisions to fundamentally remain a matter of individual clinical judgment (McNamee et al. 2015). But remarkably, this jurisdictional domain has been established in relation to a condition which does not seem to require esoteric skills. The symptoms of concussion— memory loss, dizziness, loss of consciousness—are not hard to detect, although, ironically, the condition is now claimed to be "considered among the most complex injuries in sports medicine to diagnose, assess and manage" (McCrory et al. 2013, 256). Arguably, what makes diagnosis problematic is not the specialist medical knowledge required to recognize the signs and symptoms of concussion, but the pressures experienced in the context of elite-level sport where players and coaches are highly resistant to being withdrawn from play (although studies show that schoolchildren exhibit similar non-compliance [e.g. Kroshus et al. 2015; Mrazik et al. 2015]). Consequently, the development of an essentially lay-world problem of policing injury/deviance becomes incorporated into the medical armoury, as diagnosis leads to enforced withdrawal from sport, the imposition of physical and cognitive rest, and thus the suspension of expectations of "normal" behaviour. Claims about complexity serve to justify more extensive medicalization.

Regulatory changes have progressively reinforced this process. While the initial CISG recommendation for the withdrawal of players exhibiting *any* symptoms became superseded by the less conservative emphasis on medical intervention when cases of concussion have explicitly been *diagnosed*, importantly the former was essentially amenable to lay assessment while the latter places concussion squarely within the domain of medical jurisdiction. The implementation of such guidelines further shifts the balance of jurisdictional duties between first aiders/sports trainers and physicians. Partridge (2014) notes that AFL and NRL regulations require players suspected of sustaining a concussion to be assessed by a first-aider, yet also that players "need an urgent medical assessment by a medical practitioner" because "the management of head injury is difficult for non-medical personnel" (Partridge 2014, 67, 68). Moves in various leagues to employ "concussion spotters" in the stands, or deploy an independent concussion expert to support team physicians in their concussion diagnoses, are practices premised on the belief that the complexity of concussion (as evidenced by medical uncertainty) necessitates medical monopoly.

Despite the developments which centrally position medical actors in the "solution" to concussion, there is a marked degree of subcultural resistance, which means that, of the three levels of medicalization that are potentially evident, it is at the interactional level that the process is weakest. A number of biomedical studies suggested that the reluctance to consult with medical staff (which is not unusual in sport or even in the broader population), is particularly marked in relation to athletes and brain injuries, and ascribed various reasons for this behaviour, including athletes': (a) perceptions that their condition is not serious enough, (b) reluctance to leave the game and/or let down teammates, or (c) disbelief that a concussion has occurred (Broglio et al. 2010; Fraas et al. 2013; McCrea et al. 2004). But Malcolm's (2009) study of elite rugby *explained* how attitudes towards concussion were shaped by the individual's perception that their trajectory of recovery was undetermined and could have an unpredictable impact on their lives. Athletes reported that concussions did not necessarily impair playing performance, but uncertainty over what might happen if they revealed their concerns (would they, for instance, regain their place on the team?) meant that athletes were reluctant to withdraw from sporting activities. Uncertainty also informed their decisions about whether to consult medical staff. Players knew that, in most cases, clinicians could not offer relief from symptoms or enable their recovery and return-to-play. They also knew that alerting clinical staff to their concerns about having suffered a concussion would likely only disrupt their careers and identities through enforced withdrawal from sporting activities.

More recently, Liston et al. (2018) documented athletes' distinctly risky behaviours in relation to sport-related concussions. This study of Irish amateur rugby players showed that individuals managed concussions by downplaying, ignoring, denying the significance, or concealing symptoms and "playing on." Most significantly, players spoke of their "preference" for experiencing a concussion rather than a musculoskeletal injury, arguing that the former frequently entailed a more limited impact on a person's sporting performance. They even rationalized the experiences of concussion-induced cognitive impairment as "reverting" the individual to a "primal state" and thus facilitating the kind of aggression that (many believed) contributes to rugby sporting performance. Severity of injury was assessed in relation to the length of time one was unable to play sport, and excluded considerations of longer-term neurocognitive decline. This "headstrong" attitude was derived "from within the subculture of rugby, that is, originating in the level of commitment made by players to each other and to the game" (Liston et al. 2018, 676).

The consequences of these patterns of athlete behaviour are that clinical autonomy over the management and treatment of concussion tends to be limited. Ultimately, clinicians have to negotiate the implementation of diagnostic and treatment guidelines so that they do not exacerbate patient non-compliance. Consequently, studies suggest that clinicians may seek to individualize concussions (considering how that particular player has responded to head injuries in the past) and, thus, remove diagnosis away from the necessarily generalized regulations that characterize the medicalization process (for examples, see Malcolm 2009, 2018). Alternatively, clinicians sometimes rationalize the use of their own experience to enable personal "guidelines" to supersede standardized diagnostic protocols. Both strategies effectively enable them to operationalize an understanding of concussion in ways that are most recognized and accepted by their "clients." They may, for instance, seek to avoid an explicit diagnosis of concussion and invoke alternative rationales for removing a player from play. They may, alternatively, prioritize LOC in the diagnostic criteria because their experience has shown them that this is least likely to lead to conflict with players and coaches. Ultimately, many clinicians modify their understanding of concussion and their treatment of players because their status and security in these settings cannot be guaranteed (Malcolm 2009). Through such actions, the "disunity" and incoherence of the medicalization process becomes particularly pronounced.

Conclusion

Contemporary understandings of concussion and CTE can thus be seen to have been shaped according to medicalization processes. Moreover, this "case study" illustrates how medicalization is too far-reaching and complex a process to be amenable to the control of a single unified group of medically trained individuals, or to a simple "good-bad" assessment of its consequences. Rather, medicalization must be understood as a multi-layered process which is, in many ways, uncoordinated and exhibits a combination of intended and unintended outcomes. Thus, while the medicalization of concussion (at the interactional level) is ultimately restricted due to the relative autonomy of sport as a sphere of social practice, and the relative *in*ability of medical practitioners to deliver the social value that often underpins the expansion of medicine's jurisdictional domain, it is at the same time accelerated by the longer-term and necessarily less tangible conceptual level concerns about CTE. This analysis advances previous work (e.g., Malcolm 2017) by suggesting that not only is the medicalization of concussion unevenly developed across the three respective domains, but that it is this *unevenness* that shapes our understanding and heightens social concerns. Specifically, the progression of concerns about concussion, and particularly CTE, that are being driven at the conceptual level, fuel the calls for action at the institutional and interactional level; demands which, in practice, contemporary biomedicine is unable to satisfy. As de Swaan's (1989) notion of "reluctant imperialism" suggests, the contradictions between the promise of medicine (conceptual) and the reality of delivery (institution and interactional) is not unique to this case. Medicine must continually moderate the public expectations it, in part, creates through the profession's own claims for status and influence.

But as noted earlier, none of this should be interpreted as questioning the value, or even the necessity, of medicine's presence in this field. Medicalization (at the conceptual level) has raised awareness of the potential dangers of taking part in sport, provided (at the institutional level) a more consistent set of tools with which to manage brain injuries experienced by athletes, and (at the interactional level) presents the most tangible, currently available source of help to the concussed individual. Some of these, it is increasingly well-documented, suffer considerable hardship and life-changing symptoms.

Rather, justification for the scope of existing medical interventions can be found in the degree to which the four main ethical goals of medicine are met. The *beneficence* principle of medical ethics, and the pursuit of the relief of human suffering, which is at the heart of the scientific discipline and profession of medicine, invoke a duty to attend to concerns relating to concussion and CTE. Given the potential link between combat, contact, and collision sports and both short-term neurological damage and longer-term neurocognitive decline, an element of medicalization is to be welcomed.

Against this must be a concern about the *non-maleficence* (or "first do no harm") principle of medical ethics, for whilst medical understanding of concussion and CTE remains largely exploratory, there is a danger that in certain cases the curtailment of a sphere of athletes' social or professional lives, which they find particularly meaningful and valuable, is unnecessary. Indeed, it has been argued that sports injuries in general (and, thus, concussions in particular) are experienced as particularly biographically disruptive and therefore subjectively highly problematic (Malcolm and Pullen 2018; also see Bridel et al. in this volume). Far from suggesting that the influence of medicine over the social experience of concussion has been negative, the principle of beneficence would be greatly enhanced by a broader recognition of the harm routinely done through sports participation.

Thirdly, fundamental questions also need to be raised about *equality*, for one potential outcome of the debates around concussion and CTE is to consign the health "benefits" of taking part in these activities to the most socially privileged. If, for instance, medicalization leads to the regulation of sports such that participation is only allowed where a specified (and probably costly) healthcare provision is available, then this set of activities may become restricted to the economic elite. Such exclusionary activities would, in all likelihood, become a further resource of cultural capital, which dominant social classes use to reinforce the existing social hierarchy.

Finally, and perhaps most ethically challenging of all, is the principle of *autonomy*. The resistance of sports organizations to the implementation of changes to the way sports are played cannot simply be dismissed as "ostrich-like," head-in-the-sand behaviour as portrayals such as *League of Denial* suggest (Fainaru-Wada and Fainaru 2013). While some sports organizations have reacted to proposed rule changes with an apparent ignorance of the histories of the activities which they govern (histories which show that continuous development is the normal state of affairs), equally critics must recognize that considerable justification is normally required to limit the practice of cognizant individuals capable of giving informed consent for actions which will not harm anybody but themselves. A significant consequence of medicalization may be to undermine the autonomy of individuals to take part in activities which may represent considerable risk of harm to themselves, but which they judge to represent a tangible and significant enhancement of their own life conditions. Despite such longstanding and compelling evidence linking boxing and neurocognitive decline, a fairly compelling ethical distinction (boxing is the only sport where concussion—or loss of consciousness—is a deliberate and fundamental part of competition) and substantial medical support for prohibition, it should be remembered that the sport has only ever been banned in a small minority of countries. More radical regulatory change across a wider range of sports cannot be expected until a more extensive, coherent, and compelling medicalization process has occurred.

References

Ahmed, O., and E. Hall. 2017. "'It Was Only a Mild Concussion:' Exploring the Description of Sports Concussion in Online News Articles." *Physical Therapy in Sport* 23: 7–13.

Bachynski, K. 2019. "'The Duty of Their Elders'—Doctors, Coaches, and the Framing of Youth Football's Health Risks, 1950s-1960s." *Journal of the History of Medicine and Allied Sciences*, 1–25.

Beamish, R., and I. Ritchie. 2006. *Fastest, Highest, Strongest: A Critique of High Performance Sport*. London: Routledge.

Broglio, S., Vagnozzi, R., Sabin, M., Signoretti, S., Tavazzi, B., and G. Lazzarino. 2010. "Concussion Occurrence and Knowledge in Italian Football (Soccer)." *Journal of Sports Science and Medicine* 9: 418–430.

Caron, J., Bloom, G., Johnston, K., and Sabiston, C. 2013. "Effects of Multiple Concussion on Retired National Hockey League Players." *Journal of Sport & Exercise Psychology* 35: 168–179.

Castellani, R., and G. Perry. 2017. "Dementia Pugilistica Revisited." *Journal of Alzheimer's Disease* 60 (4): 1209–1221.

Conrad, P. 1992. "Medicalization and Social Control." *Annual Review of Sociology* 18: 209–232.

Conrad, P. 2007. *The Medicalization of Society: On the Transformation of Human Conditions into Treatable Disorders*. London: Johns Hopkins University Press.

Conrad, P. 2015. "Foreword." In *Reimagining (Bio)medicalization, Pharmaceuticals and Genetics: Old Critiques and New Engagements*, edited by S. Bell, and A.E. Figert, vii–ix. London: Routledge.

Craton, N., and O. Leslie. 2014. "Time to Re-think the Zurich Guidelines? A Critique on the Consensus Statement on Concussion in Sport, Held in Zurich, November 2012." *Clinical Journal of Sports Medicine* 24 (2): 93–95.

De Swaan, A. 1989. "The Reluctant Imperialism of the Medical Profession." *Social Science and Medicine* 28 (11): 1165–1170.

Fainaru-Wada, M., and Fainaru, S. 2013. *League of Denial*. New York: Crown Business.

Fox, R.C. 2000. "Medical Uncertainty Revisited." In *The Handbook of Social Studies in Health and Medicine* edited by G.L. Albrecht, R. Fitzpatrick, and S.C. Scrimshaw, 409–425. London: Sage.

Fraas, M., Coughlan, G., Hart, E., and C. McCarthy. 2013. "Concussion History and Reporting Rates in Elite Irish Rugby Union Players." *Physical Therapy in Sport* 15: 136–142.

Halfmann, D. 2011. "Recognizing Medicalization and Demedicalization: Discourses, Practices and Identities." *Health* 16 (2): 186–207.

Hardes, J. 2017. "Governing Sporting Brains: Concussion, Neuroscience, and the Biopolitical Regulation of Sport." *Sport, Ethics & Philosophy* 11: 281–293.

Harrison, E. 2014. "The First Concussion Crisis: Head Injury and Evidence in Early American Football." *American Journal of Public Health* 104: 822–833.

Hillman, A., and J. Latimer. 2017. "Cultural Representations of Dementia." *PLOS Medicine* 14 (3): e102274.

Hoberman, J. 1992. *Mortal Engines: The Science of Performance and the Dehumanization of Sport*. New York: Free Press.

Illich, I. 1975. *Medical Nemesis*. London: Calder & Boyers.

Kroshus, E., Garnett, B., Hawrilenko, M., and C. Baugh. 2015. "Concussion Under-Reporting and Pressure from Coaches, Teammates, Fans and Parents." *Social Science and Medicine* 134: 66–75.

Kuhn, A., Yengo-Kahn, A., Kerr, Z., and S. Zuckerman. 2017. "Sports Concussion Research, Chronic Traumatic Encephalopathy and the Media: Repairing the Disconnect." *British Journal of Sports Medicine* 51: 1732–1733.

Liston, K., McDowell, M., Malcolm, D., Scott, A., and I. Waddington, I. 2018. "On Being 'Head Strong': The Pain Zone and Concussion in Non-Elite Rugby Union." *International Review for the Sociology of Sport* 53 (6): 668–684.

Malcolm, D. 2006. "Unprofessional Practice? The Power and Status of Sports Physicians." *Sociology of Sport Journal* 23 (4): 376–395.

Malcolm, D. 2009. "Medical Uncertainty and Clinician-Athlete Relations: The Management of Concussion Injuries in Rugby Union." *Sociology of Sport Journal* 26 (2): 191–210.

Malcolm, D. 2013. *Globalizing Cricket: Englishness, Empire and Identity.* London: Bloomsbury.

Malcolm, D. 2015. "Elias and the Sociology of Sport." In *Routledge Handbook of Sociology of Sport,* edited by R. Giulianotti, 50–60. London: Routledge.

Malcolm, D. 2017. *Sport, Medicine and Health: the medicalization of sport?* London: Routledge.

Malcolm, D. 2020. *The Concussion Crisis in Sport.* London: Routledge.

Malcolm, D., and E. Pullen. 2018. "'Everything I Enjoy Doing I Just Couldn't do': Sport-related Injury and Biographical Disruption." *Health: An Interdisciplinary Journal for the Social Study of Health, Illness and Medicine.* http://journals.sagepub.com/doi/pdf/10.1177/1363459318800142

Malcolm, D., and A. Scott. 2011. "Professional Relations in Sport Healthcare: Workplace Responses to Organisational Change." *Social Science and Medicine* 72: 513–520.

McCrea, M., T. Hammeke, G. Olsen, P. Leo, and K. Guskiewicz. 2004. "Unreported Concussion in High School Football Players: Implications for Prevention." *Clinical Journal of Sports Medicine* 14: 13–17.

McCrory, P. 1999. "You Can Run but You Can't Hide: The Role of Concussion Severity Scales in Sport." *British Journal of Sports Medicine* 33: 297–280.

McCrory, P. 2001. "When to Retire after Concussion?" *British Journal of Sports Medicine* 35: 81–82.

McCrory, P., W. Meeuwisse, M. Aubrey, et al. 2013. "Consensus Statement on Concussion in Sport: The 4th International Conference on Concussion in Sport held in Zurich, November 2012." *British Journal of Sports Medicine* 47: 250–258.

McGannon, K., S. Cunningham, and R. Schinke. 2013. "Understanding Concussion in Socio-Cultural Context: A Media Analysis of a National Hockey League Star's Concussion." *Psychology of Sport and Exercise* 14: 891–899.

McNamee, M., B. Partridge, and L. Anderson. 2015. "Concussion in Sport: Conceptual and Ethical Issues." *Kinesiology Review* 4: 190–202.

Mez, J., D.H. Daneshvar, P.T. Kiernan, et al. 2017. "Clinicopathological Evaluation of Chronic Traumatic Encephalopathy in Players of American Football." *Journal of the American Medical Association* 318 (4): 360–370.

Mrazik, M., C. Dennison, B. Brooks, K.O. Yeates, S. Babul, and D. Naidu. 2015. "A Qualitative Review of Sports Concussion Education: Prime Time for Evidence-Based Knowledge Translation." *British Journal of Sports Medicine* 49: 1548–1553.

Parsons, T. 1975. "The Sick Role and the Role of the Physician Reconsidered." *The Millbank Memorial Fund Quarterly* 53 (3): 257–278.

Partridge, B. 2014. "Dazed and Confused: Sports Medicine, Conflicts of Interest, and Concussion Management." *Bioethical Inquiry* 11: 65–74.

Sharp, D., and P. Jenkins. 2015. "Concussion is Confusing Us All." *Neurology* 15: 172–186.

Sheard, K. 1998. "'Brutal and Degrading': The Medical Profession and Boxing, 1838–1984." *International Journal of the History of Sport* 15 (3): 74–102.

Sheard, K. 2003. "Boxing in the Western Civilizing Process." In *Sport Histories: Figurational Studies of the Development of Modern Sports*, edited by E. Dunning, D. Malcolm and I. Waddington, 15–30. London: Routledge.

Shurley, J., and J. Todd. 2012. "Boxing Lessons: An Historical Review of Chronic Head Trauma in Boxing and Football." *Kinesiology* 1: 170–184.

Stewart, W., Allinson, Al-Sarraj, S. et al. 2019. "Primum non Nocere: A Call for Balance When Reporting CTE." *Lancet Neurology* 18: 231–232.

Sullivan, S., A. Schneiders, C. Cheang, E. Kitto, H. Lee, J. Redhead, et al. 2012. "'What's happening?' A Content Analysis of Concussion-related Traffic on Twitter." *British Journal of Sports Medicine* 46: 258–263.

Ventresca, M. 2019. "The Curious Case of CTE: Mediating Materialities of Traumatic Brain Injury." *Communication and Sport* 7 (2): 135–156.

Waddington, I. 1996. "The Development of Sports Medicine." *Sociology of Sport Journal* 13 (2): 176–196.

Waddington, I., and P. Murphy. 1992. "Drugs, Sport and Ideologies." In *Sport and Leisure in the Civilizing Process*, edited by E. Dunning, and C. Rojek, 36–64. London: Macmillan.

Weinberg, S.K., and H. Around. 1952. The Occupational Culture of the Boxer." *American Journal of Sociology* 62: 460–469.

Williams, S.J., C. Coveney, and J. Gabe. 2018. "The Concept of Medicalisation Reassessed: A Response to Joan Busfield." *Sociology of Health and Illness* 39 (5): 775–780.

Wilson, J. 2019 "Premier League Players to Assist in Research into Concussion." *The Daily Telegraph*, January 16. www.telegraph.co.uk/football/2019/01/16/ premier-league-players-assist-research-concussion/

Workewych, A., M. Muzzi, R. Jing, S. Zhang, J. Topolovec-Vranic, and M. Cusimano. 2017. "Twitter and Traumatic Brain Injury: A Content and Sentiment Analysis of Tweets Pertaining to Sport-related Brain Injury." *SAGE Open Medicine* 5: 1–11.

Zola, I. 1983. "Medicine as an Institution of Social Control." *Sociological Review* 20 (4): 487–504.

3 "A Clear Conscience"

Advertising Football Equipment and Responsibility for Injuries[1]

Kathleen Bachynski

In 1905, the *Washington Post* asserted that whereas football was once "a diluted" English game with "little real meat to it," the sport had rapidly transformed into an American pastime. As evidence, the newspaper claimed that one factory was churning out twenty times more football supplies than it had five years prior. Now American cities might have two uniformed football teams on average, the *Post* estimated. Undoubtedly, manufacturers had "clothed more ambitious youngsters with canvas jackets this year than they ever have before." Football's remarkable popularity was a "common truth" that every sporting goods dealer in the United States "cheerfully granted" (Football Old Game 1905).

It was no coincidence that the *Post* framed the rapid development and expansion of football in terms of uniformed teams, factory output, and the cheers of sporting goods dealers. The proliferation of equipment in many ways defined the American sport emerging at the turn of the twentieth century. The production of standardized sporting goods, in conjunction with a "network of expert coaches, journalists, administrators, manufacturers, and dealers," was increasingly demarcating the boundaries of organized athletics (Hardy 1990).

Protective equipment and its makers also shaped public perceptions of youth football's physical risks, especially with regard to traumatic brain injuries. Manufacturers' advertisements and their responses to product liability cases were particularly influential, in sometimes contradictory ways. In advertisements, manufacturers needed to portray football as sufficiently risky to require extensive protective gear but not so dangerous that the purchase of pads and helmets could not minimize the harms. In addition, advertisements throughout the twentieth century associated equipment with desirable social values for boys, such as personal fulfillment, athletic achievement, confidence, and the ability to aspire to future football careers at higher levels of play.

Yet in defending themselves against product liability lawsuits, which typically focused on helmets and head injuries, manufacturers emphasized the lack of relationship between their products and the injuries of individual plaintiffs. Manufacturers further argued that individual coaches, parents, and children should take responsibility for preventing injuries because they had voluntarily chosen to assume the risks of the sport. They threatened that lawsuits would doom football by rendering sports equipment manufacturing and insurance prohibitively costly. Ultimately, manufacturers largely succeeded in framing the issue of football safety as a matter of individual responsibility while presenting protective equipment as necessary and sufficient to address safety concerns. Developed over decades, this approach has continued to influence understandings of how to address youth sports concussions through the early twenty-first century.

Advertising Equipment

Sports marketing and management researchers have argued that in the 1920s, sporting goods advertisements shifted from promoting product quality to more intangible appeals. This is consistent with analyses of marketing strategies in other industries. For example, Kodak did not stress the superior luminescence of its photographic film but rather highlighted the promise and satisfaction of memories preserved. Similarly, sports advertisements increasingly emphasized how equipment could enhance personal style, identity, and fulfillment (Fielding and Miller 1996, 37–50; Levitt 1981, 94–102).

Advertisements for protective gear, however, inherently signaled to consumers that sports carried a certain element of risk. The importance of communicating that equipment could minimize those risks thus interacted with the emphasis on personal fulfilment and achievements. For decades, sporting goods manufacturers consistently promoted their equipment to athletes and coaches as both protecting players against injuries as well as improving athletic performance.

For example, a 1935 advertisement for Rawlings football equipment entitled "Banish fear of injuries" was published in *Athletic Journal,* a trade journal aimed at coaches. The subsequent text emphasized that without fear of getting hurt, athletes could play tougher. "Your men can smash through and play their hardest when outfitted with Rawlings equipment. . . . They'll buck, tackle and block with that air of confidence born only through banishment of injury fears" (Rawlings 1935). The Wilson Sporting Goods Company told coaches that "the ability of your team to win" depended on the action, protection, and comfort afforded by their lines of football equipment (Wilson 1935). Their gear included saddle seat football pants, cantilever shoulder pads, corset-back helmets, thigh guards, and kidney pads that were built to cover players' hip bones, kidneys, pelvic bones, and lower ribs. The J.A. Dubow Manufacturing Company observed that while good football equipment alone couldn't win championships, by preventing injuries and giving players assurance, quality equipment was a key part of the "victory complex" (J. A. Dubow 1935).

Such advertisements not only communicated that football equipment could minimize risks, but that eliminating injury concerns was crucial to athletic achievements. In so doing, equipment ads promoted ideals of toughness associated with particular forms of twentieth century American masculinity.

Beliefs about male physical aggression were reinforced by a number of medical and educational authorities who stressed that boys inherently needed physical contact that only full-body collision sports like football could provide. For example, in 1931 team physician Joseph H. Burnett wrote that properly supervised football "gives boys a natural outlet for their nervous energies and keeps them off the streets" (Burnett 1931, 32). On this view, if boys could not "smash through" one another in adult-supervised sports, they might find a more socially threatening outlet for their inherent drives. Protective gear facilitated athletic aggression while purportedly shielding players from its harmful physical consequences.

Advertisements aimed both at coaches and prospective athletes promulgated remarkably similar claims through the decades. Sales pitches to younger players included an additional appeal that child athletes could emulate their older role models. Such ads became more common in the 1950s, when prepubescent boys increasingly began playing organized football. For example, in 1959 Rawlings published an advertisement featuring NFL coach Buddy Parker that targeted young prospective football players. Pictured next to a young boy wearing a football helmet, Parker recommended Rawlings equipment, explaining that the manufacturer's helmets and shoulder pads not only protected against injury, "but they give the confidence and freedom of action needed for good blocking and tackling." The ad further noted that Parker and the players named in the advertisement were members of Rawlings' advisory staff. An additional portion of the ad promoted a "Tobin Rote helmet" and a "Bobby Layne official youth football," both named for professional football stars of the day (Rawlings 1959).

This advertisement had appeared in *Boys' Life*, the official youth magazine of the Boy Scouts of America. *Boys' Life*, which had a circulation of over 500,000 in the early 1950s and 2.4 million by 1967, was an attractive venue for manufacturers seeking to reach young readers (Do Boy Scouts Rate 1967, 73–74). Even when advertisements lacked the explicit sponsorship of professional coaches or players, messages targeted at younger boys emphasized that the equipment would afford youth athletes the same protection as their older football heroes. In the September 1960 issue of *Boys' Life*, for example, MacGregor depicted a boy wearing a football helmet and a reproduction of a Baltimore Colts uniform, "just like the pros wear!" (MacGregor 1960, 78). Meanwhile, Wilson asked young readers if they were ready for big-time football, stating that "Wilson gives you the same type of protective equipment worn by leading high school, college, and professional teams. You get the same helmet and pads worn by top gridiron stars, scaled to your size to give you maximum protection." Football equipment was a means by which children in youth leagues could aspire to future high school, college, and even professional football stardom. Pads and helmets were thus imbued with many meanings, from eliminating fear of injuries to enabling boys to identify with football heroes and allowing them to see themselves on the path to similar athletic achievements (Wilson 1961, 42–43).

In addition to linking their equipment with athletic role models, sporting goods manufacturers studied how to make the best use of boys' relationships with their family, particularly their fathers. In 1958, the Institute for Motivational Research examined sales, advertising, and merchandising challenges for the Rawlings Sporting Goods Company (Institute for Motivational Research 1958). The Institute was an advertising consultancy firm whose founder would later be dubbed "the patron saint of motivational research" (Rothenberg 1989; Stern 2004). The Institute's study devoted much space to developing a "typology of paternal participants" and how the company could craft its appeals accordingly. The study was primarily focused on baseball gloves, but the report suggested that its findings could be applied to Rawlings' other product lines, and even that the company should emphasize "the continuity of sports in all seasons" by offering packages including, for instance, a baseball glove, a basketball, and a football (Institute for Motivational Research 1958).

The report identified three types of fathers, each of whom could provide a particular target for advertising appeals. The first was the "vicarious athlete," who sought to recapture his own athletic past and participated in athletics through his son. The vicarious athlete perceived the best equipment as enabling his son to perform well. Secondly, the "genuine athlete" believed in the value of sports participation as an integral part of a "healthy life." Finally, the "indifferent athlete" was a father whose primary interest was in developing a strong relationship with his child. He was thus drawn to sports not as a good in itself but as an instrument to strengthening a father-child relationship. Identifying these relationships as key to sporting goods purchases, the report recommended that Rawlings craft appeals to each of these types of fathers. For example, to appeal to the "indifferent athlete" father, Rawlings could produce advertisements that depicted fathers and sons in action, enjoying sports together (Institute for Motivational Research 1958).

The October 1955 cover of *Boys' Life* magazine depicted this idealized relationship between fathers and sons playing football, with an added twist: the two sons and father on the cover mirrored the positions of the professional football players seen on their living room television (see Figure 3.1). Interestingly, the two sons wore football headgear, but not their father. This likely indicates that youth football was already associated with the organized version of the game that required protective equipment. Fathers, on the other hand, were perceived as informally "roughhousing" with their sons. The *Boys' Life* scene reinforced the importance of protective gear for youth. Helmets protected vulnerable boys from injuries and enabled them to aspire to future athletic success. Tellingly, the father's college football trophies and photos appear on a nearby shelf. This imagery, both in equipment advertisements and boys' magazines, illustrated how male role models, from professional players to fathers, could promote the desirability of youth football participation.

Advertisements also featured numerous and longstanding claims about the scientific design of equipment, although no standards for football helmets or other protective football equipment existed before the 1970s. For

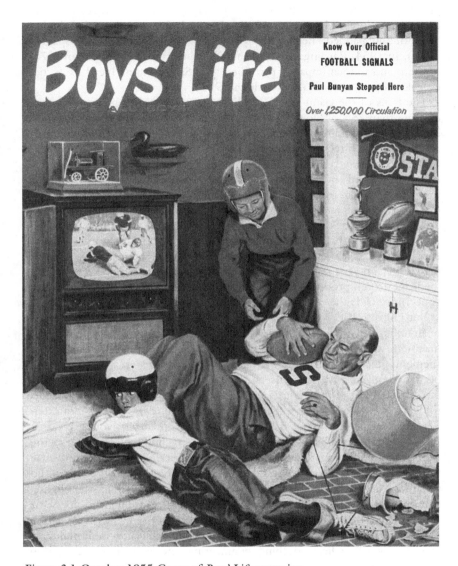

Figure 3.1 October 1955 Cover of *Boys' Life* magazine.

Source: Image by cover artist Carol Johnson. © *Boys' Life* magazine/Boy Scouts of America.

example, in 1932, the Witchell Sheill Company advertised its "scientific football shoes" featuring "eleven points of superiority" (Witchell Sheill Company 1932). In 1946, Brooks Shoe Manufacturing Company promoted its "scientifically constructed shoes," which would "positively" prevent football injuries (Brooks Shoe 1946). In 1947, MacGregor Goldsmith described its new plastic football helmet as "the product of many years' painstaking research and experimentation" (MacGregor 1947, 17). In 1950, Spalding advertised its "scientifically padded" helmet to provide the "utmost" protection (Spalding 1950). In 1954, Rawlings asserted that its helmet could dissipate "over 75% of sharp and sudden impact," providing "the Safest, Surest Head Protection ever developed for football" (Rawlings 1954).

The basis of the claim that a Rawlings helmet could dissipate the impact of more than 75% of blows to players' heads is unclear. Yet many unsourced but scientific-sounding statements persisted in decades of football equipment advertising. Such techniques were certainly not limited to sports equipment. Claims promoting "scientific design," undocumented statistics about product effectiveness, and endorsements from experts were common features of many forms of American advertising in the twentieth century. Perhaps most notoriously, the tobacco industry used images and endorsements from physicians to claim that cigarettes would improve consumer health (Gardner and Brandt 2006). Many football advertisements similarly drew on American confidence in scientific research and laboratory design to promote their products. In making such claims, manufacturers invoked the prestige of scientific research and medicine to sell products that addressed a broad range of health and safety concerns outside the control of organized medicine (Tomes 2001).

But unlike tobacco manufacturers, whose advertisements masked the risks of an unhealthy product associated with chronic disease, sporting goods manufacturers were promoting products intended to prevent injuries. Their advertisements implicitly, and often explicitly, acknowledged that football could be dangerous activity. Advertisers of protective gear thus had to portray a nuanced portrait of the hazards associated with collision sports: they needed to depict youth football as sufficiently risky to require the purchase of extensive equipment, but not so risky as to be inappropriate for young children. Protective equipment ads communicated that technology and engineering were effective in mitigating risks, and often specifically emphasized manufacturers' alliances with coaches and doctors in working to protect children. For instance, a 1951 Rawlings ad for rubber-plastic football helmets highlighted that the headgear "complies fully with the safety recommendations of the American Football Coaches Association, doctors and trainers, *AND* is built with Rawlings [*sic*] half-century of 'know-how'." Such claims indicated that a combination of medical, coaching, engineering, and manufacturing expertise informing the design of protective gear afforded the greatest possible protection (Rawlings 1951).

Product Liability and the Limitations of Helmets

Advertisements communicated that technology was effective in mitigating significant physical risks and in empowering boys to play an aggressive collision sport safely and confidently. Yet in defending themselves against product liability lawsuits, manufacturers took a different approach. They instead emphasized the lack of relationship between their products, particularly helmets, and the injuries of individual plaintiffs. Although advertisements were an important driver of public expectations of helmet safety, in legal settings, manufacturers instead highlighted the limitations of equipment.

Sports injury lawsuits had not always been a common occurrence for potentially vulnerable parties, such as school districts, coaches, and sporting goods manufacturers. Through the 1960s, courts typically applied a legal doctrine known as "assumption of risk." This principle held that athletes playing competitive sports knowingly and voluntarily assumed the risks by choosing to participate, and could not recover from sports-related harms. As a result, the limited lawsuits resulting from sports injuries typically found plaintiffs responsible for assuming the risks (Drago 2002).

The case of *Vendrell v. School District No. 26C, Malheur County* exemplifies the application of this doctrine. In 1953, then-fifteen-year-old high school football player Louis Vendrell suffered a broken neck after being tackled by two members of the opposing team. In his testimony, Vendrell recalled that after he saw the other team's players in front of him, "I knew I couldn't go any further so I put my head down and just ran into em [*sic*] and that is when I heard my neck snap." The injury resulted in permanent paraplegia. In his suit against the school district, Vendrell claimed that he had not received "proper or sufficient instructions" in the techniques of football, nor had he been provided "the necessary and proper protective equipment" (Thornton et al. 2012, 136).

Vendrell's case reached the Supreme Court of Oregon in 1962. But the court found neither his football coaches nor the school district negligent. In its reasoning, the court explained that no prospective football players, including children, needed to be warned that they might sustain an injury. While not explicitly characterizing permanent paralysis itself as an inherent part of the game, the court nonetheless indicated that coaches did not have a duty to warn athletes of potential injuries, because no warning should be necessary:

> Body contact, bruises, and clashes are inherent in the game. There is no other way to play it. No prospective player need be told that a participant in the game of football may sustain injury. That fact is self-evident. It draws to the game the manly; they accept its risks, blows, clashes and injuries without whimper. No one expects a football coach to extract from the game the body clashes that cause bruises, jolts and hard falls. To remove them would end the sport.
>
> (Vendrell v. School District No. 26C 1962, 412–413)

The court's reasoning reframed boys as adults; indeed, the court's very language suggested that the essence of football was to attract "the manly" and transform boys into men. The risks of football, and the willingness to sustain these injuries "without whimper," were treated as inherent components of this vision of masculinity. Removing those risks "would end the sport," a scenario the court's language presented as flatly unacceptable. The court further dispensed with Vendrell's argument that his coaches had not taught him to avoid using his head, stating that "one of the first lessons that an infant learns when he begins to toddle about on his feet is not to permit his head to collide with anything." Vendrell was thus found to have assumed all the risks of tackling. These risks were so obvious, the court indicated, that even infants ought to be aware of the potential dangers of subjecting one's head to blows (Vendrell v. School District No. 26C 1962, 412–413).

Such rulings meant that even catastrophically injured child athletes were unlikely to find success in the courtroom. But in 1963, the Supreme Court of California held in *Greenman v. Yuba Power Products, Inc.* that manufacturers would face strict liability for injuries to human beings caused by defects of their products. This new standard of strict liability meant that plaintiffs would not need to prove negligence or intent to cause injury, only that the product had caused a person harm. Strict products liability quickly swept across the United States, a change one leading tort law scholar described as "the most rapid and altogether spectacular overturn of an established rule in the entire history of the law of torts" (Prosser 1966, 791–848). Courts would go on to recognize three general types of manufacturer conduct that might make a product unsafe: defective design of product, defective manufacture of product, and inadequate marketing or failure to warn (Abraham 2008; Gershonowitz 1987; Graham 2014; Prosser 1966).

The move toward strict liability made sporting manufacturers increasingly vulnerable to lawsuits. Plaintiffs contended that manufacturers had a duty to warn consumers that helmets could not protect against particular head and brain injuries. For instance, in 1974, a Texas high school football quarterback, Mark Daniels, sustained a head injury in a collision with a teammate. The force of the impact resulted in an indentation in his helmet. Daniels, subsequently diagnosed with a subdural hematoma that left him with severe and permanent brain damage, sued Rawlings Sporting Goods. The 20th Judicial District Court of Robertson County, Texas, awarded Daniels a $1.5 million judgment, a decision which Rawlings unsuccessfully appealed. In upholding this ruling, Texas' 10th District Court of Appeals explained that while all evidence suggested that the primary purpose of a helmet was to protect its wearer against head and brain injuries, nonetheless:

> Defendant [Rawlings] admitted that it never made any attempt to warn potential users of the limitations of its helmets; that it had known for a long time that helmets will not protect against brain injuries; that it made the "conscious decision" not to tell people the helmet would not protect against subdural hematomas; that the company "elected" not to warn that the helmets would not protect against head injuries, in spite of the knowledge that laymen believe that the purpose of the helmet is to protect the head.
>
> (Rawlings Sporting Goods Co., Inc. v. Daniels 1981)

The court's assertion that Rawlings consciously chose not to warn consumers of its helmets' limitations could be considered the promotion of ignorance as a strategic ploy on the part of the manufacturer. As historian Robert Proctor has argued, ignorance is not necessarily "natural," but instead can be deliberately fostered in order to advance particular interests. The question of what knowledge manufacturers possessed, and what information they chose to divulge to or withhold from consumers, was at the crux of this and similar legal cases (Proctor 2008).

Stead v Riddell and the American Way of Sport

In addition to arguing that manufacturers needed to warn of the inherent limitations of helmets, plaintiffs also contended that manufacturers should be held liable for defective helmet designs. One such suit, *Stead v. Riddell*, emerged as a landmark case to which both manufacturers and lawyers would point as representing trends in product liability law. In numerous settings, from congressional hearings to medical journals, these groups deployed *Stead v. Riddell* to advance their preferred framing of the legal responsibility for youth football injuries.

Greg Stead was paralyzed from the neck down due to an injury he sustained on the opening kickoff of a 1971 high school football game. In 1975, Stead sued Riddell, one of the most prominent football helmet manufacturers, contending that the improper design of the helmet had contributed to his catastrophic injury. His attorney argued that after a player on the opposing team kicked Stead, causing his client's head to jerk backward, Stead's neck was broken between the fourth and fifth vertebrae by the unpadded back of the Riddell helmet he was wearing. By the time of the trial, Stead was 20 years old and sat through the five-week proceedings in a wheelchair. He won his case: a jury awarded Stead $5.3 million in damages (Helmet Maker 1975; Dupree 1977, D1).

Sporting goods manufacturers and their lawyers depicted *Stead v. Riddell* as heralding an impending wave of lawsuits that threatened their ability to do business. A Riddell lawyer would later characterize this 1975 case as the beginning of an "onslaught" of damage suits filed against helmet manufacturers (Sports People 1984). Although the multimillion-dollar award was unusual, *Stead v. Riddell* was certainly consistent with a broader legal trend of courts increasingly imposing liability on manufacturers. Examining products liability law through 1990, two legal scholars found that beginning in the mid-1970s through the early 1980s, courts "seemed to compete with each other to see who could make it easiest for plaintiffs to reach juries with claims of defective product design" (Henderson and Eisenberg 1990, 484).

Manufacturers turned to *Stead v. Riddell* as the perfect example of litigation run amok in their advocacy efforts to minimize their susceptibility to such suits. Notably, in 1976, the SGMA formed the Multi Association Action Committee (MAAC) to address product liability. The committee included

119 leaders from a range of industries beyond sporting goods manufacturing, such as aircraft, cast metals, recreation vehicles, and small farm implements. The stated goals of MAAC included: "to call attention to the plight of industry manufacturers in product liability suits and costs for defense" and "to notify Americans that we have unleashed a wave of unfounded suits and attendant unprecedented awards that guarantee inflation for the next decade" (underline in original) (MAAC 1976, 3).

At MAAC's SMGA-sponsored conference on liability reform in 1976, SGMA president Harold J. Bruns referenced the Stead case. "Did you know that a football helmet manufacturer lost a $5.3 million lawsuit to an injured player while the defendant's attorney contended there was no proof that the injured party was even wearing the defendant's helmet?" Bruns asked. He further alluded to Stead's presence in the courtroom throughout the trial as unjustly swaying the jurors against the manufacturers. Although jurors were charged to render decisions based on fact and fairness, Bruns complained, they "instead must view a paraplegic in a wheelchair which conjurs [*sic*] irresistible emotion and remorse." Consequently, "a sports equipment manufacturer is made to pay a fortune out of sympathy rather than neglect." Depicting such cases as frivolous and opportunistic, Bruns suggested that justice was being "outwitted by lucid trial lawyers." Manufacturers were forced to pay extravagant sums as "a sacrifice to ease the social conscience." Bruns hastened to clarify that he was certainly not blaming "the paraplegic doomed to a life of thinking," nor the judges and juries doing what they believed to be right. Instead, he contended that the legal system was at fault (Bruns 1976, 95–97).

Bruns urged reform of the tort system as the ultimate solution. In 1977, he explained to the *Chicago Tribune* that the SGMA's goal was to return the law of the land "back to where it was prior to 1964, when the doctrine of strict liability was adopted" (Husar 1977). In the testimony he submitted to the U.S. Senate's Select Committee on Small Business, Bruns laid out specific actions and reforms the SGMA sought: public awareness of the problem, statute of limitations on manufactured products, limitation of awards, plaintiff to assume responsibility for all defendant's costs related to unfounded suits, limitation on contingency fees, state of the art at time of manufacture as a defense, and elimination of punitive damages. He threatened that if the product liability crisis were not abated, "next year may well be the last year for the Super Bowl." The notion that lawsuits threatened the very existence of football would persist in the SGMA's policy arguments through the 1980s and early 1990s (Bruns 1976, 20).

The vision of lawsuits extinguishing football was also repeatedly disseminated at conferences and in journals aimed at sports medicine specialists. "The whole existence of contact sports as we know them is being threatened," said one speaker at the 1977 annual meeting of the American College of Sports Medicine (Husar 1977). A 1985 *Physician and Sportsmedicine* article promulgated the view that manufacturers had made football helmets safer, and as a "reward," they had become subjected to increasing legal liability for football injuries (Tally 1985). This analysis highlighted the toll such lawsuits were taking on manufacturers, casting the sporting goods manufacturers as victims of multimillion-dollar lawsuits. A 1987 article in the *Physician and Sportsmedicine*, whose very title signaled the dangers to "the American way of sport," opened with the image of a high school football game under way in "Anytown, United States." The author, a contributing editor of the journal, suggested that this scene, "as American as apple pie," might be in danger of disappearing. She cited sporting goods manufacturers as a source of the concern. Sports medicine physicians, whose work was fundamentally tied to organized sports, were thus encouraged to share the SGMA's framing of product liability law as posing an existential threat to sports (Lubell 1987, 192–200).

The example of *Stead v. Riddell*, as well as liability concerns faced by sporting goods manufacturers more generally, also featured prominently in debates over federal legislation. In April 1976, President Gerald Ford established a Federal Interagency Task Force on Product Liability to study product liability law and ways to stabilize recoveries and insurance premiums. The task force continued its work under President Carter and ultimately recommended the drafting of a model uniform law for use by all states. The task force also recommended the enactment of federal legislation to allow small businesses to form self-insurance pools; such legislation would ultimately become law in 1981 as the Product Liability Risk Retention Act (Dworkin 1981; Schwartz and Behrens 1996).

But before the passage of this act, in 1977, the U.S. Senate held hearings to consider an earlier version of product liability legislation. The bill, proposed by senators John C. Culver (D-Iowa) and Gaylord Nelson (D-Wisconsin), would have established a national product liability insurance administration and arbitration program, as well as a product liability insurance pool (The New Insurance Crisis 1977). The perspective of manufacturers on *Stead v. Riddell* featured in these hearings in the form of letters submitted by William C. Merritt, who had defended Riddell against the lawsuit brought by Stead. Merritt's arguments illustrate how sports manufacturers sought to frame product liability lawsuits and to deflect responsibility for football injuries away from themselves.

Merritt drew on social prejudices to argue that the Florida jury that had ruled against Riddell was largely composed of "middle class people of not high intelligence" (Merritt 1977, 406). He noted the inclusion of a black maid, the wife of a civil servant, an Italian terrazzo tile man, a Cuban postal clerk, and a retired man on the jury. Not only did the judge ask questions during the *voir dire* to play upon the sympathies of these purportedly simpleminded jurors, Merritt suggested, but the judge also failed to understand the suspension system of Riddell's helmet and its irrelevance to a neck injury case. Merritt emphasized the testimony of the assistant football coach at the high school where Greg Stead had played. The coach stated that he had specifically and repeatedly instructed Stead that "you stick a man with your helmet and your [*sic*] going to break your neck" (Merritt 1977, 409).

Merritt further questioned the credibility of Harold Fenner, who had been brought in as a witness for the plaintiff. Fenner had testified that the helmet's ability to attenuate the impact of blows to the head could contribute to the plaintiff's neck injury. Merritt repeatedly emphasized that Fenner was not board certified as an orthopedic surgeon and that other experts disagreed with Fenner's assessment (Merritt 1977). "Medical research has shown that the helmet has no relationship to the injury," Merritt would continue to insist in the following years (Elich 1987). Lawyers and the sporting goods manufacturers they represented thus argued that well-meaning but relatively uneducated jurors were unduly swayed by the sympathy-inducing presence of catastrophically injured athletes; that these athletes had been sufficiently warned by their own coaches of the risk of injury; and that medical testimony about the possible role of the helmet was uncertain and suspect.

Beginning in the 1970s, a number of manufacturers ceased making football helmets. Remaining manufacturers claimed that helmet lawsuits were driving them out of business. In 1970, there were eighteen manufacturers of football helmets in the United States; by 1994, there were only two (Sullivan 1996). In 1977, Frank Gordon, the president of Riddell, told the *Chicago Tribune* that manufacturers were toying, half seriously, with the notion of "going on strike" and not producing helmets for a year or two, to draw public attention to the legal crisis. While such a strategy was not particularly realistic, suggesting the threat of a football helmet manufacturing strike to a major American newspaper was in itself a means of raising public concern (Husar 1977). A *Los Angeles Times* article claimed that "making football helmets can be as potentially risky as playing the game without any" (Sing 1979).

While manufacturers blamed product liability laws, consumer groups including the National Insurance Consumer Organization, the Consumer Federation of America, and Public Citizen contended that insurers were charging exorbitant premiums to compensate for poor risk judgments in previous years. The president of the National Insurance Consumer Organization told the *New York Times* that while the courts had expanded the concept of liability, that had nothing to do with insurance rates. "The insurance problem shouldn't be used as an excuse to take away victims' rights to sue" (Lewin 1986).

Despite—or perhaps thanks to—the emphatic alarm that sporting goods manufacturers continued to sound in the press, in legislative hearings, and in medical journals, ultimately not many multimillion-dollar cases were settled in favor of plaintiffs. In fact, in 1979, the chief financial officer of Wynn's International Inc., which had recently acquired Riddell, observed that despite a spate of lawsuits following *Stead v. Riddell*, "since then, we have not had any large adverse jury awards or large settlements." He characterized *Stead v. Riddell* as an "anomaly" (Sing 1979). In fact, by the late 1980s, the legal trend was instead moving toward limiting plaintiffs' rights to recover damages for product-related injuries. Two legal scholars suggested that this "quiet revolution in products liability" might be attributed to the success of tort reformers in linking product liability cases to the insurance crisis of the mid-1980s. In the area of athletic equipment, they found that plaintiffs had a success rate in two-thirds of cases from 1979–1984, which decreased to less than half of cases in 1985–1989 (Eisenberg and Henderson 1992).

Individual Responsibility for Football Injuries

But perhaps the manufacturers' most notable strategy was their argument that the fundamental responsibility for football injuries should rest with players, their parents, and coaches. This argument fit in with broader, prevailing American beliefs about individual responsibility for addressing health problems. For instance, in an influential 1977 article, physician and president of the Rockefeller Foundation John Knowles argued that educating individuals about health risks, from cigarettes to lack of exercise, and promoting a culture which encouraged individuals to assume responsibility for their behaviors, were the key to improving health. By making legal arguments that emphasized the personal responsibility of individual child athletes and parents to assume the risks of football, sporting goods manufacturers drew on these beliefs about who should be held responsible for health problems (Knowles 1977).

An SGMA-funded coalition advanced this perspective in a strategy reminiscent of other industry-sponsored front groups. In 1990 hearings before the U.S. Senate, the SGMA described their public education operation, the Coalition of Americans to Protect Sports (CAPS), as being founded in 1986 as "a grassroots organization whose purpose is to inform coaches, schools, and the general public about the detrimental impact liability is having on manufacturers of sports equipment and programs across the United States" (SGMA 1990, 595). Rather than a broad-based grassroots movement, however, CAPS was primarily an arm of the SGMA. Lobbyist Richard Feldman recalled that in 1988, he and other SGMA leaders renamed the group CAPS in order to make it sound more like a united national organization (Feldman 2007, 136).

As part of its goal to minimize the potential for liability litigation, CAPS asserted that better equipment and personal responsibility would address the issue of safety in sports. For instance, Sharon Lincoln, the communications director of CAPS, argued that lawsuits discouraged people "from accepting the rational, logical, and foreseeable risks of their own behavior." She singled out football as essential to American culture and education. Lincoln argued that although football was particularly vulnerable to liability lawsuits and thus more costly to play and to insure, "many school administrators would laugh at the idea of doing away with it. Football is financially critical to schools." Instead of filing lawsuits, players and coaches needed to accept the risks and take responsibility for preventing them. CAPS developed a risk education program aimed at sports administrators and coaches that emphasized the ways such "nonsensical" lawsuits could be avoided (Lincoln 1992, 40–42, 63).

In the *Journal of Physical Education, Recreation & Dance*, Lincoln promoted the *CAPS Sports Injury Risk Management Manual* and other CAPS materials "to help the sports community maximize athlete safety while minimizing the potential for litigation. . . . CAPS provides a checklist of safety precautions for coaches to follow and can update them on some of the most common types of sports accidents resulting in litigation, as well as the frivolous, nonsensical cases that pull coaches and school districts away from their teams and into the courtrooms." CAPS artwork included an image of a dejected youth baseball player sitting under a sign that read, "Field closed due to lack of insurance." These materials were disseminated in manuals, videos, and clinics (Lincoln 1992, 40–42, 63).

Similar to the public relations strategy of big tobacco companies and fast-food industry groups of shifting responsibility for risk away from themselves and onto consumers, CAPS sponsored a vision of individual responsibility for the health risks of competitive sports (Friedman, Cheyne et al. 2015). CAPS presented their safety strategies as essential for avoiding lawsuits and high insurance premiums that threatened the existence of youth sports. In the form of educational resources to protect sports and the health of players, the SGMA shared a message of personal responsibility for safety that obscured the involvement of industry interests.

A Clear Conscience

Manufacturers would continue to invoke safety claims in equipment advertisements, conveying a reassuring sense of scientific design and product effectiveness. As one high school football coach, a self-described "safety kook," put it in 1984, "I feel that if every kid has his equipment checked by a professional, if something happens to the kid, I'll have a clear conscience" (Sperling 1984). But when confronted with legal claims, manufacturers instead underscored the limitations of their equipment and their lack of responsibility for injuries sustained by consumers. The function of equipment in providing reassurance—and absolution in the event of injury—highlights one of the most important ongoing tensions in the debates over protective football equipment: whether even the best equipment can effectively compensate for the limits of the human body.

As they continue to claim their products will both protect athletes and enhance performance, sporting goods manufacturers continue to influence public beliefs about the relationship between football equipment and player safety. In response to heightened concussion concerns of the 2010s, manufacturers such as Riddell have marketed their helmets as offering player protection and head impact monitoring technology (Riddell 2014). These campaigns have contributed to broader sports industry efforts to frame such strategies as better helmet design and education campaigns as sufficient to alleviate football's risks (Bachynski and Goldberg 2014). Indeed, in response, parents and athletic directors have sought the most advanced, state-of-the-art protective equipment to continue to allow children to play tackle football. The executive director of the National Operating Committee on Standards for Athletic Equipment told the *New York Times* that sales of football helmets had dramatically changed since 2011. "I see high school athletic directors submitting purchase orders for 500 five-star helmets. Parents are saying, 'I don't want a four-star helmet, I want the best for my kid'" (Klein 2014).

Simultaneously, manufacturers continue to highlight the limitations of helmets in court settings to protect themselves legally. Notably, in 2013, parents and players filed a class-action lawsuit against Riddell, charging that the manufacturer had put forward misleading claims that their helmets could reduce the risks of concussions. In response, Riddell lawyers pointed to disclaimers placed within helmets emphasizing that no helmet could prevent brain injuries or concussions (Zambito 2015). On this view, it remains up to players and families to purchase the most advanced equipment possible while taking individual responsibility for brain injuries on the gridiron. Through advertisements and legal arguments that have absolved many sports stakeholders of responsibility for injury, manufacturers continue to profoundly shape youth football and American ideas about risk, masculinity, and concussions.

Note

1. Adapted from Bachynski, Kathleen. 2019. *No Game for Boys to Play: The History of Youth Football and the Origins of a Public Health Crisis.* Chapel Hill, NC: University of North Carolina Press. Copyright by University of North Carolina Press. Reprinted with Permission.

References

Abraham, Kenneth S. 2008. *The Liability Century: Insurance and Tort Law from the Progressive Era to 9/11.* Cambridge, MA: Harvard University Press.

Bachynski, Kathleen E., and Daniel S. Goldberg. 2014. "Youth Sports & Public Health: Framing Risks of Mild Traumatic Brain Injury in American Football and Ice Hockey." *The Journal of Law, Medicine & Ethics* 42 (3): 323–333.

Brooks Shoe Manufacturing Company. 1946. "Brooks Safety Football Shoes." *Scholastic Coach* 15: 35.

Bruns, Howard J. 1976. "Statement on Product Liability." In *Proceedings of the MAAC Liability Reform Conference*, 95–97. Washington, DC, September 7–8.

Bruns, Howard J. 1978. "Testimony for Select Committee on Small Business, U.S. Senate." In *Proceedings of the MAAC Liability Reform Conference,* 20–23. Washington, DC, September 7–8.

Burnett, Joseph H. 1931. "Survey of Football Injuries in the High Schools of Massachusetts." *Journal of Health and Physical Education* 2 (8): 32–33, 50.

"Do Boy Scouts Rate a Badge for Retailing?" *Business Week,* August 12, 1967, 73–74.

Drago, Alexander J. 2002. "Assumption of Risk: An Age-Old Defense Still Viable in Sports and Recreation." *Fordham Intellectual Property, Media and Entertainment Law Journal* 12 (2): 583–608.

Dupree, David. 1977. "Sports Equipment on Trial." *Washington Post,* December 31.

Dworkin, Terry Morehead. 1981. "Product Liability Reform and the Model Uniform Product Liability Act." *Nebraska Law Review* 60 (1): 50–80.

Eisenberg, Theodore, and James A. Henderson, Jr. 1992. "Inside the Quiet Revolution in Products Liability." *UCLA Law Review* 37: 731–810.

Elich, Patricia. 1987. "Butting Heads: Miami Lawyer Carl Rentz Tackles the Country's Biggest Helmet Manufacture." *The Sun-Sentinel*, February 16.

Feldman, Richard. 2007. *Ricochet: Confessions of a Gun Lobbyist*. Hoboken, NJ: John Wiley & Sons.

Fielding, Lawrence W., and Lori K. Miller. 1996. "Advertising and the Development of Consumer Purchasing Criteria: The Sporting Goods Industry, 1900–1930." *Sports Marketing Quarterly* 5 (4): 37–50.

"Football Old Game: Gridiron Sport Was Introduced Thirty Years Ago," *The Washington Post*, October 8, 1905.

Friedman, Lissy C., Andrew Cheyne, Daniel Givelber, Mark A. Gottlieb, and Richard A. Daynard. 2015. "Tobacco Industry Use of Personal Responsibility Rhetoric in Public Relations and Litigation: Disguising Freedom to Blame as Freedom of Choice." *American Journal of Public Health* 105 (2): 250–260.

Gardner, Martha N., and Allan M. Brandt. 2006. " 'The Doctors' Choice is America's Choice': The Physician in US Cigarette Advertisements, 1930–1953." *American Journal of Public Health* 96 (2): 222–232.

Gershonowitz, Aaron. 1987. "The Strict Liability Duty to Warn." *Washington and Lee Law Review* 44 (1): 71–107.

Graham, Kyle. 2014. "Strict Products Liability at 50: Four Histories." *Marquette Law Review* 98 (2): 555–624.

Hardy, Stephen. 1990. " 'Adopted by All the Leading Clubs': Sporting Goods and the Shaping of Leisure, 1800–1900." In *For Fun and Profit: The Transformation of Leisure Into Consumption*, edited by Richard Butsch, 71–101. Philadelphia: Temple University Press.

"Helmet Maker Must Pay $5.3m to Injured Player." *Boston Globe*, December 12, 1975.

Henderson, Jr., James A., and Theodore Eisenberg. 1990. "The Quiet Revolution in Products Liability: An Empirical Study of Legal Change." *UCLA Law Review* 37: 479–553.

Husar, John. 1977. "Liability Suits Threaten Helmet Makers." *Chicago Tribune*, June 5.

Institute for Motivational Research, Inc. 1958. A Motivational Research Pilot Study of the Sales, Advertising, and Merchandising Problems of Rawlings Sporting Goods. Croton-on-Hudson, NY: Institute for Motivational Research, Inc.

J.A. Dubow Manufacturing Company Advertisement. 1935. "Dubow: What will the Year Bring Forth????" *Athletic Journal* 16 (1): 45.

Klein, Jeff Z. 2014. "Spartan Hockey Helmets Going Under Microscope." *New York Times*, July 22. www.nytimes.com/2014/07/23/sports/hockey/for-safety-hockey-helmets-going-under-microscope.html.

Knowles, John H. 1977. "The Responsibility of the Individual." *Daedalus* 106 (1): 57–80.

Levitt, Theodore. 1981. "Marketing Intangible Products and Product Intangibles." *Harvard Business Review* 59 (3): 94–102.

Lewin, Tamar. 1986. "The Liability Insurance Spiral." *New York Times*, March 8.

Lincoln, Sharon M. 1992. "Sports Injury Risk Management & the Keys to Safety." *Journal of Physical Education, Recreation & Dance* 63 (7): 40–42.

Lubell, Adele. 1987. "Insurance, Liability, and the American Way of Sport." *The Physician and Sports Medicine* 15 (9): 192–200.

MAAC. 1976. *Proceedings of the MAAC Liability Reform Conference.* Washington, DC, September 7–8. Sponsored by the Sporting Goods Manufacturers Association; publisher not identified.

MacGregor Advertisement. 1960. "Just Like the Pros Wear!" *Boys' Life*, September, 78.

MacGregor Goldsmith Advertisement. 1947. "Game-Tested and Proven." *Scholastic Coach*, September, 17.

Merritt, William C. 1977. "Re: *Stead* v. *Riddell, Inc.*, Claim No.: 010787 267 71 55, D/A: September 30, 1971, Our File No: 75–252 WCM." In *Product Liability Insurance Hearings before the Subcommittee for Consumers of the Committee on Commerce, Science, and Transportation*, 406–413. United States Senate, Ninety-fifth Congress, first session, on S. 403, April 27, 28, and 29.

"The New Insurance Crisis." *Washington Post*, February 24, 1977.

Proctor, Robert. 2008. "Agnotology: A Missing Term to Describe the Cultural Production of Ignorance (and Its Study)." In *Agnotology: The Making and Unmaking of Ignorance*, edited by Robert Proctor, and Londa Shiebinger, 1–33. Stanford, CA: Stanford University Press.

Prosser, William L. 1966. "The Fall of the Citadel (Strict Liability to the Consumer)." *Minnesota Law Review* 50: 791–848.

Rawlings Advertisement. 1935. "Banish Fear of Injuries." *Athletic Journal* 15 (8): no page.

Rawlings Advertisement. 1951. "Defense Against Injury!" *Athletic Journal* 31 (1): inside front cover.

Rawlings Advertisement. 1954. "Rawlings Triple Protection Head Cushion." *Scholastic Coach* 23: 3.

Rawlings Advertisement. 1959. "Here's How to Start Playing Football Right!" *Boys' Life* September: 8.

Rawlings Sporting Goods Co., Inc. v. Daniels.1981. 619 S.W.2d 435 (Tex.Civ.App.).

Riddell Newsroom. 2014. "New Riddell Speedflex Highlights the Future of Football Helmet Design and Innovation." *Riddell Press Release*, August 26. http://news.riddell.com/info/releases/new-riddell-speedflex-highlights-the-future-of-football-helmet-design-and-innovation.

Rothenberg, Randall. 1989. "Advertising; Capitalist Eye on the Soviet Consumer." *New York Times*, February 15.

Schwartz, Victor E., and Mark A. Behrens. 1996. "The Road to Federal Product Liability Reform." *Maryland Law Review* 55 (4): 1363–1383.

SGMA. 1990. "Statement of the Sporting Goods Manufacturers Association." *Product Liability Reform Act: Hearings Before the Subcommittee on the Consumer of the Committee on Commerce, Science, and Transportation*, 595–597. United States Senate, One Hundred First Congress, Second Session, on S. 1400, February 22, April 5, and May 10.

Sing, Bill. 1979. "Helmet Making Perilous as Football." *Los Angeles Times*, October 8.

Spalding Advertisement. 1950. "Here's the Helmet with the Big Safety Margin." *Athletic Journal* December: 17.

Sperling, Michael. 1984. "Uniforming a Football Team is Complex, Costly Procedure." *Washington Post*, August 16.

"Sports People; Damaging Lawsuits." 1984. *New York Times*, December 9. www. nytimes.com/1984/12/09/sports/sports-people-damaging-lawsuits.html.

Stern, Barbara B. 2004. "The Importance of Being Ernest: Commemorating Dichter's Contribution to Advertising Research." *Journal of Advertising Research* 44 (2): 165–169.

Sullivan, Shea. 1996. "Football Helmet Product Liability: A Survey of Cases and Call for Reform." *Sports Lawyers Journal* 3: 233–260.

Tally, Jean. 1985. "Reward for Increasing Football Helmet Safety? Legal Hassles." *The Physician and Sportsmedicine* 13 (2): 161–168.

Thornton, Patrick K., Walter T. Champion, Jr., and Lawrence S. Ruddell. 2012. *Sports Ethics for Sports Management Professionals*, 136. Sudbury, MA: Jones & Bartlett Learning.

Tomes, Nancy. 2001. "Merchants of Health: Medicine and Consumer Culture in the United States, 1900–1940." *The Journal of American History* 88 (2): 519–547.

Vendrell v. School District No. 26C, Malheur County. 1962. 376 P. 2d 406, 412–413.

Wilson Advertisement. 1935. "Wilson Offers You Advanced Equipment at a Price to Fit Your Budget." *Athletic Journal* 15 (8): 28–29.

Wilson Advertisement. 1961. "Are You Ready for Big-Time Football Equipment?" *Boys' Life* September: 42–43.

Witchell Sheill Company Advertisement. 1932. "Witchell Scientific Football Shoes." *Proceedings of the Twelfth Annual Meeting of the American Football Coaches Association*. New York, December 27–28.

Zambito, Thomas. 2015. "Judge's Ruling Puts Football Helmet Lawsuit Back in Play." *NJ.com*, August 4. www.nj.com/news/index.ssf/2015/08/judge_rules_football_helmet_lawsuit_back_in_play.html.

4 Football Helmet Safety and the Veil of Standards

Daniel R. Morrison

Introduction

As the editors point out in their introduction to this volume, public concern about concussion, and the challenge this presents to players, coaches, and sports industries at all levels of play is perhaps at an all-time high (e.g., Feudtner and Miles 2018; Ventresca and McDonald, this volume). Nowhere is this concern more evident, and the stakes higher, than in American football. The issues are complex, with multiple stakeholders and layers of analysis available. Media reports document the link between participation in tackle football and brain injuries like concussion (e.g., Mariano and Peebles 2017). Research interest in concussions, sub-concussive brain injuries, and the cumulative effects of head impact exposure on youth and college players is high (Bachynski 2016; Daniel et al. 2012; Papa et al. 2018). In addition to the biomechanical issues involved, some scholars have argued that National Football League (NFL) funding of public health research into football-related brain injury represents a significant conflict of interest that must be addressed (Bachynski and Goldberg 2018).

Concern among athletes, families of youth players, and other stakeholders about the relationship between collision sports like football and brain injury has generated renewed interest in football helmet design. Discussion has focused on the goal of making equipment that prevents concussions and sub-concussive injuries, and that may reduce the incidence of longer-term outcomes such as CTE. Research on football helmets and their effectiveness in preventing brain injuries has a long history. Harrison (2014) documents change in headgear, from simple stocking caps for team identification to more recent plastic helmets that are designed to prevent skull fracture. She argues that advocates tied football to core American values, framing the game's inherent risks as manageable, even as physician and public awareness of football-related concussion grew from the late nineteenth century into the early twentieth (Harrison 2014). Today, public and scientific attention remain focused on the promise and peril of football helmets for protecting players' brains from concussion and other injuries.

Consider these contrasting headlines: "This May Be the Helmet that Solves Football's Concussion Crisis" (Fuhrmeister 2014) and "High-tech Helmets Won't Solve the NFL's Concussion Problem" (McFarling 2019). The first article profiles Riddell's updated helmet technology and research that quantifies the number and severity of hits to the head. The second argues that even the most expensive helmets (such as the VICIS Zero1 and Riddell's form-fitting model) do not protect players any better than less expensive models. Both articles illustrate the enduring interest in reducing risks to player health by technological means.

This focus on helmet technologies and their role in mitigating risk to brain health amount to what Bachynski and Goldberg (2014) call a "technological imperative." The technological imperative "refers to the general belief in the significance of technology to human progress in general, and to American progress in particular" (2014, 328). Football helmets and the technology behind them have significant symbolic power in the debate over the link between concussion, sub-concussive blows, and longer-term brain health. Helmets serve as a kind of cultural keystone, materially binding together concern about brain health, controversies over injury causation, and deeply held values said to be embodied by American football (Taylor et al. 2019). Complex cultural debates indeed converge through the design, manufacture, and testing of football helmets.

Sociologists of knowledge, sports, and public health should be interested in the controversy that concussion science presents because scholars in each field have unique perspectives from which to understand the issues; indeed, each field is likely to present a number of interesting, interlocking questions. Sociologists of knowledge might ask how and for whom science is mobilized in documenting the prevalence of concussive and sub-concussive head injuries; how scientists construct causal pathways from injury to disease and injury to impairment; or examine how "sound science" is variously mobilized within the controversy over brain injury in collision sports.

For scholars in public health, questions about the prevalence of these injuries, their long-term consequences, adequate equipment, and the precautionary principle are all relevant. The precautionary principle states, "Where there are threats of serious or irreversible damage, lack of full scientific certainty shall not be used as a reason for postponing cost-effective measures [for prevention]" (Stirling 2007). Goldberg suggests that if there is any significant risk of permanent neurological damage by playing football, then changing the rules and equipment may be both ineffective and inefficient steps to protect short- and long-term health (Goldberg 2013). What if the precautionary principle leads us to the conclusion that no football helmet can sufficiently protect players from concussion? Full-contact practices and game conditions will still inherently expose players to collisions associated with both concussion and sub-concussive brain injuries.

In this chapter, I identify a gap in the existing literature, namely, the missing analysis of how private, non-profit standards-setting organizations influence the design and testing of sports equipment such as football helmets. I introduce a new concept, "the veil of standards," to investigate how current safety standards conceal scientific uncertainty regarding the likelihood of concussion in football. Interrogating the work performed by standards and standardization processes in creating inequities in the distribution of socially valuable knowledge, I argue that this veil simultaneously creates knowledge for equipment makers and other officials while producing ignorance for others. In this case, standards are one important way powerful groups like equipment makers and trade groups can downplay and may conceal the possibility of long-term damage to a player's brain. The veil of standards separates those groups with more privileged access to scientific knowledge and uncertainty from those with less access such as players, youth player parents, and some coaches. In this case, standards-setting bodies are pivotal actors in creating and maintaining the veil.

To build my case, I offer empirical material from the National Operating Committee on Standards for Athletic Equipment (NOCSAE), the American standards-setting body for football helmets, focusing on recent revisions to standardized testing procedures and performance standards for helmets. NOCSAE specifies testing methods and performance measures for newly manufactured and recertified football helmets. Coinciding with increased public scrutiny and intense media coverage of sports brain injuries, NOCSAE has revised these standards within the last five years. Standard performance specifications for newly-manufactured helmets were revised in January, February, and July of 2017, and then modified again in July 2018 and January 2019 (NOCSAE 2019b). Although originally scheduled for implementation in July 2018, implementation of these revised standards has been pushed back three times, and is (at the time of this writing) now set for November 2019. The major change behind these new standards is the addition of measures of rotational acceleration via pneumatic ram test. Although not yet implemented, these new standards for youth and adult football helmet performance seemingly respond to neuroscientific and biomechanics research demonstrating the importance of both linear and rotational acceleration as mechanisms for brain injuries such as concussion. I argue that NOCSAE's safety standards can mislead players and their families about the degree of protection provided by football helmets while the organization disavows responsibility for both acute and longer-term injuries that may occur during normal use. I offer a pragmatic, sociological account of standards and standardization, focusing on the epistemic disadvantages and inequality that operate in this field.

This chapter proceeds as follows. First, I review recent work in the sociology of science and knowledge that theorizes the social production of ignorance. This work analyzes the production of ignorance through an analysis of scientific agenda-setting: the process communities of scientists decide which questions to take up in their research. Understanding the role of agenda-setting is essential for answering questions about how scientific knowledge is produced, for which audiences, and for what purposes. Agenda-setting is a key mechanism where knowledge and lack of knowledge about football helmets is simultaneously produced. I couple this with a discussion of the precautionary principle from Stirling (2007), who unpacks the relationship between igno-rance, uncertainty, ambiguity, and risk. Then, I explain how the production of ignorance and processes of agenda-setting occur through current NOCSAE standards and describe mandated helmet-testing procedures. In this section, I suggest that current safety standards produce knowledge for the preven-tion of skull fracture but do little to address what is known about concussion and sub-concussive brain injuries. The chapter continues with an analysis of the NOCSAE standards scheduled to come into effect in November 2019 and suggests that testing procedures used in these revised standards may still be inadequate to address the biomechanical mechanisms for concussion. This chapter concludes with a summary of preceding points and suggestions for future research using the "veil of standards" concept. Such research would help scholars interrogate the many ways that standards and standardization processes contribute to epistemic inequality, defined as socially significant gaps in an individual or collective's stock of knowledge.

Scientific Agenda-Setting and the Production of Knowledge

A growing number of sociologists, anthropologists, and philosophers are ask-ing important questions about research agendas that produce some forms of knowledge but not others. These scholars ask us to consider how research agendas simultaneously reveal and conceal knowledge (McGoey 2012). Fric-kel asks, "Why are certain kinds of scientific knowledge created, certified, and circulated while other kinds are not?" (2014b, 263). Critiquing the dominant tradition in the sociology of scientific knowledge that focuses on the construc-tion and stabilization of scientific facts, he writes, "we have not cultivated a tradition of systematically tracking the consequences of the non-production of knowledge" (Frickel 2014b, 265). Frickel charges his readers to consider the obverse side of discovery, the creation of non-knowledge. For example, knowledge gained by designing football helmets that prevent skull fractures is different from, and may be counterproductive for, the goal of preventing concussion and/or sub-concussive injuries. Scholars such as Frickel invite us to consider the structure of ignorance and "undone science" alongside the structure of scientific knowledge. Both, he argues, are socially produced through individual scientist and field-level decision-making processes that set the agenda for research, including some questions and research programs but not others (see also Frickel et al. 2010; Hess 2016).

Several authors offer complex renderings and typologies of ignorance, non-knowledge, and knowledge absence (e.g., Croissant 2014; Rappert and Bauchspies 2014). Andrew Stirling's early work offers much needed clarity, connecting these issues to public policy through the precautionary principle. In his article about risk and the precautionary principle in science, Stirling

(2007) distinguishes between two essential parameters necessary to assess risk. The first is knowledge about a set of events that may happen, such as, "hazards, possibilities or outcomes" (2007, 309), the likelihood that these things will happen, and the probability of their occurrence. Contrasting more or less complete forms of knowledge of what events may happen and their likelihood gives Stirling (2007) four potential states of incomplete knowledge: risk, uncertainty, ambiguity, and ignorance.

The concept of risk, Stirling argues, should be used to describe situations in which knowledge about possibilities and their probabilities is most complete. In these situations, we are both able to specify what outcomes are possible and the likelihood that any one or more will actually happen. For example, if we know that car accidents occur, and we know the probability of any one car being involved in an accident, then we can, on average, determine how risky driving a car on any given day would be. In contrast, uncertainty is defined as having knowledge of types of outcomes, but lack of clarity regarding the probability of each outcome. Uncertainty is most likely to accompany complex and open systems, human elements in causal models, unassessed carcinogens, and the like (Stirling 2007). In these cases, it is impossible to calculate the probability of a particular outcome. Stirling notes that, when uncertain, the best approach is, "to acknowledge various possible interpretations . . . under uncertainty, attempts to assert a single aggregated picture of risk are neither rational nor 'science-based'" (2007, 310). Acknowledging differences of interpretation and the inability to reasonably assess risk should encourage researchers, policy makers, and others to approach such situations with caution, seeking input from a broad community of stakeholders.

Ambiguity is defined by known probabilities but unknown outcomes, accompanying events that are certain to occur or that have already happened, but whose outcomes are unclear are thus defined as ambiguous. Stirling suggests that ecological, safety, and social criteria of harm are all ambiguous in this way. When the outcomes are ambiguous, we must not seek final analysis of risk but rather conduct further inquiry (Stirling 2007). Ignorance, however, is defined as the state in which neither probabilities nor outcomes can be specified. Neither the full range of outcomes possible, nor the probabilities of their occurrence, are fully known (Stirling 2007). Ignorance thus makes risk assessment untenable and supports the wisdom of the precautionary principle. For example, outcomes from climate change were unknown, and the probability of each event unclear. As scientists' work in climate science advanced, ignorance decreased and more sophisticated risk assessment became possible (Stirling 2007). With this advancement came clarification of outcomes and probabilities, but new questions—with their attendant uncertainties and ambiguities—developed as well.

Applying these ideas to football helmets means assessing the state of knowledge regarding outcomes—in this case, concussion, sub-concussive injuries, and longer-term consequences such as CTE—and their probabilities. Although research has been conducted on the likelihood of concussion in NCAA and NFL, estimates vary widely. For example, Houck and colleagues examined nine years of medical records for one NCAA Football Bowl Subdivision team (Houck et al. 2016). These researchers found that of the 452 unique players on the roster, 26% sustained a concussion. Examining two years of NFL data, Lawrence et al. reported a concussion rate of 27.8 per 1,000 athletes at risk (Lawrence et al. 2015). Despite the widespread public and scientific interest in the connection between exposure to tackle football and degenerative brain conditions such as CTE, challenges remain. Research in this area has been hampered by the fact that CTE can be diagnosed only by direct examination of the brain post-mortem. This remains the case, even as new research evaluates the possibility of testing for tau-protein levels in the brain via PET (positron emission tomography) scan (Belson 2019).

A recent study by Boston University researchers suggests that closed-head impacts may lead to CTE without evidence of concussion (Tagge et al. 2018). Reacting to recent evidence from a convenience sample that found evidence of CTE in 99% of former professional football players, Binney and Bachynski (2019) estimated that CTE prevalence in the cohort of 1,142 former NFL players who died between February 2008 and May 2016 ranges from 9.6% to near 100%. They thus argue that CTE prevalence in this group of NFL players is significant despite selection effects (2019).

Responses to this research have varied considerably, and a great deal is at stake. Other scholars, including authors for this collection, note the profitability of the sport for its owners and the lucrative contracts negotiated by the NFL. For example, in their book *League of Denial*, Mark Fainaru-Wada and Steve Fainaru (2013) document the entanglement of big-time sports, big money, and brain health science. They argue that the NFL's early efforts to understand the link between football and brain injury were led by inexperienced doctors with incentives to protect the game and its profitability over the health and safety of athletes (see also Bachynski and Goldberg 2018). Other NFL-funded efforts have been stopped by the league due to concerns over inaccurate sensor technology in helmets (Davidson 2015). Although UNC-Chapel Hill football coach Larry Fedora was widely criticized when he questioned the causal connection between football and CTE (Chuck 2018), some neuropsychologists continue to deny or downplay the link between football and long-term brain injury (Solomon 2018). Other advocates call for more protective measures and have turned to enhancing helmet technology in an effort to better protect players' brains.

The most recent evidence illustrates that we do know *something* about the brain health outcomes that are possible in collision sports like football in the short-term (concussion and sub-concussive injuries) and longer-term (CTE, dementia, behavioral problems, and others). What we do not know is how likely these outcomes are, and which players are most likely to experience them (Binney and Bachynski 2019). Following Stirling's typology, the science is in a state of ambiguity.

If concussion science is in a state of ambiguity, then it is likely football players and those who purchase football helmets may share that state—knowing that concussions are a problem, but unaware of how likely any participating player is to experience one or more of these injuries. It may then be productive to ask: for whom is this ambiguity beneficial and who might be harmed? Which groups stand to gain from the lack of clarity in the specific mechanisms of concussive injury and ambiguity around the role football helmets could play in prevention? Although some research has documented a disconnect between societal outcomes, such as prevention, and private-sector agendas, including profits (Wallace and Ràfols 2018), little has been done to apply such an analysis to the world of safety standards in athletics. In what follows, I examine how NOCSAE, a private, non-profit standards-setting organization, shapes debate over football helmet safety, their standards operating to veil or restrict access to knowledge that may be valuable for players, coaches, trainers, youth parents, and, ultimately, the fate of the game itself as we learn more about the mechanisms of football-related brain injuries.

Football Helmet Safety and the Veil of Standards

NOCSAE plays a significant, if under-recognized, part in shaping both public perception and scientific inquiry into the relationship between tackle football and brain injuries. According to their website, "NOCSAE is an independent and nonprofit standards development body with the sole mission to enhance athletic safety through scientific research and the creation of performance standards for athletic equipment" (NOCSAE 2019a). Indeed, head and neck injuries, and associated fatalities, spurred the creation of NOCSAE in 1970 (NOCSAE n.d.-b). NOCSAE focused in its early years on ways to reduce fatalities and other career-ending injuries through setting standards for football helmets (NOCSAE n.d.-b). By 1973, NOCSAE adopted its first set of football helmet safety standards, and fatalities on the football field have since declined dramatically. This private, non-profit body's 19-member board of directors includes representatives from organizations such as the American College of Sports Medicine, the American Society for Sports Medicine, the National Athletic Trainers' Association, the American Academy of Pediatrics, the American Football Coaches Association, and the National Collegiate Athletic Association, among others (NOCSAE 2018b). NOCSAE's composition and leadership—an executive director, research grants director, and technical director—is important because it illustrates the extent to which certain stakeholder groups are part of the core group while others, such as parents of youth players and adult players themselves, are not included (NOCSAE n.d.-a).

A NOCSAE Standards Committee is responsible for developing, reviewing, and modifying helmet standards. NOCSAE's public statements do, however, tout the group's commitment to openness and public engagement. Their "Overview" document, for example, states, "The standards development process is open to the public, and participation by any interested party is encouraged and facilitated through public meetings and extended comment periods" (NOCSAE 2018b). Public commitment to an open process may help maintain NOCSAE's legitimacy, because the group invites stakeholders not formally included in committees or on the board of directors. The standards, once developed, influence which helmets are made and how they are marketed to consumers.

NOCSAE limits its involvement in the equipment industry to discussing, revising, and publishing standards that manufacturers must meet to qualify for the NOCSAE seal, which is then affixed to each approved helmet. Helmet testing is conducted by private contractors, rather than NOCSAE itself. Despite its limited role in the helmet manufacturing and certification process, however, NOCSAE's standards are very powerful. Compliance with NOCSAE standards by equipment manufacturers and re-conditioners (companies who refurbish used equipment) is technically optional, but in practice is virtually mandatory since the standards have been adopted by every major sports association in the United States and many abroad (NOCSAE 2018b). Helmets not meeting NOCSAE standards are essentially banned from the market, since they are prohibited by all major sporting bodies. NOCSAE standards, then, have significant influence on the design of football helmets and serve as an important constraint for designers. While related to NOCSAE, public-facing ratings such as Virginia Tech's STAR system do not directly challenge existing standards. Rather, the STAR system summarizes the results of a correlation between head impacts experienced through one season of play and results from NOCSAE-style drop tests (Rowson and Duma 2011). The STAR system includes data from on-field head impacts and in-laboratory testing, with the goal of more accurately measuring differences between NOCSAE-approved helmet models.

Until recent testing further restricted player choice, helmets were only minimally regulated by and within the NFL. In 2012, a *New York Times* journalist reported that the league deemed any NOCSAE certified helmet appropriate for use by its players, irrespective of its performance on more rigorous safety trials (Borden 2012). Laboratory research jointly funded by the NFL and the NFL Players Association rated 34 helmets and resulted in the banning of 10 out of the 34 helmets tested. Six helmets performed so poorly that they were banned immediately in 2018, while four were permitted for use by players who had worn them in the previous season and prohibited entirely for all new players (NFLPA 2018). One of the game's highest-profile players, Tom Brady, was allowed to keep wearing his helmet during the 2018–2019 season even though it had been prohibited under the league's new regulations (Vrentas 2018). The NFL now prohibits some NOCSAE-certified helmets, signaling the inadequacy of the current standards. This move demonstrates that NOCSAE standards and mandated testing procedures reveal only certain aspects of helmet performance in regard to protection against impact and thus restrict other potential tests and associated metrics that may provide better information and more helpful ratings.

Standards, and the standardized testing procedures that verify compliance, are intended to provide a level playing field for manufacturers and to ensure that each helmet model is assessed using identical conditions and test procedures every time. Since standards, by definition, are about enforcing a certain level of quality, they also raise conceptual issues about what is concealed and revealed by their use. A performance benchmark is a binary, either-or outcome that conceals how well each helmet tested and the differences in performance between helmets that meet NOCSAE standards. NOCSAE addresses these limitations by indicating that, since the test is rigorous, all helmets must score substantially less than the 1,200 severity index score, which is a measure of the protective qualities of the helmet, in order to pass (NOCSAE 2018a).

Just how much each helmet can be expected to reduce the likelihood of concussion, sub-concussive blows, and potentially, significant brain disease, is systematically unknown in current testing procedures mandated by NOCSAE. Indeed, this question is effectively ruled out by the standards themselves. Altogether, NOCSAE's standards, the testing regime, and the public display of these standards represents a clear example of what I call the veil of standards. In this case, a private, non-profit association of groups interested in selling football helmets and managing perceptions of football's inherent risks, such as equipment manufacturers and representatives of major sports organizations, work to define helmet safety standards (see also Bachynski and Goldberg 2018). These standards function, in part, by creating inequities in the distribution of socially valuable knowledge. The veil of standards operates as the dividing line between front and backstage operations (Goffman 1959). Like Goffman's backstage region, the work of creating a group of interested parties, working through competing proposals for testing standards, piloting those standards, promulgating them, and ensuring compliance, is blackboxed behind the veil of standards. My claim, then, is that the veil of standards obscures the process of knowledge production while it guides safety research. The veil of standards operates in a curious way here: it ensures a baseline of "safety" for athletic equipment for the public while simultaneously downplaying the politics of safety standards to these same consumers and fans. Just how the veil of standards works in everyday testing practices is explained in the next section.

The Drop Test and the Perils of Rotational Force

NOCSAE mandates that samples of each helmet model be subjected to 26 drop tests from varying heights (and thus varying impacts), 6 from standard front, right-front, side, right rear, rear, and top positions, the remaining tests conducted on random positions (NOCSAE DOC ND 001–17m17b, 2017). The tests are conducted in both normal heat (approximately 72 degrees Fahrenheit) and high heat (100 degrees Fahrenheit). Inside each of three bio-mimicking headforms, a sensor detects the amount of force generated by each impact. Each headform simulates different-sized players. The helmet sits on an articulating "neck" and is usually tested without a faceguard. These straight-ahead impacts are the only ones currently required by NOCSAE, despite the widespread consensus that both linear and rotational forces are present in real-world football collisions and cited in a review of concussion biomechanics (Duma and Rowson 2014).

NOCSAE's standard test method for athletic headgear is described in 33 pages, which include references, a list and definitions of terms, sampling procedures, recertification requirements, and a summary of modifications since January 2015 (NOCSAE DOC ND 001–17m17b, 2017). Written for technical specialists at certified testing locations such as NOCSAE Technical Director David Halstead's Southern Impact Research Center (NOCSAE n.d.-a), this lengthy document constitutes a barrier to non-specialist understanding of testing requirements and contributes to the veil of standards. Although NOCSAE's own materials boast of more than 150 updates to football standards, the most significant updates are arguably due to the recent addition of pneumatic ram tests for rotational acceleration, which are described below (NOCSAE 2018a).

Similar procedures are used for Virginia Tech's STAR ratings. Unlike NOCSAE's standard, however, Virginia Tech's first rating system was based on a metric that summarized 24 drop tests along with the proportion of head impacts each football player can expect to experience throughout a season (Rowson and Duma 2011). Virginia Tech's assessment drops helmets from between 12 and 60 inches, with peak impact forces from 0 g to over 140 g at 60 inches. As with the NOCSAE example, helmets are dropped on one of four locations six times each, for a total of 24 impacts. This STAR rating work is more sophisticated because it used the HIT (Head Impact Telemetry) System to record impacts wirelessly from six in-helmet accelerometers. Recognizing that not all players experience the same number of head impacts while on the field, the HIT protocol attempted to measure the number and strength of impacts received by player helmets. When a player was hit, impact data was recorded, transmitted wirelessly, and assessed (Daniel et al. 2012; Rowson and Duma 2011).

Despite the widespread use of NOCSAE standards, and the use of a similar system by leading helmet safety scientists at Virginia Tech, the inadequacy of modeling linear impacts in assessing concussion risk is well-known. For example, the Institute of Medicine's 2014 report on sports concussions and youth stated, "current testing standards and rating systems for protective devices do not incorporate measures of rotational head acceleration or velocity and therefore do not comprehensively evaluate a particular device's ability to mitigate concussion risk" (Institute of Medicine and National Research Council 2014, 11). Dr. Robert Cantu, a Boston University neurosurgeon and founding member of the Concussion Legacy Foundation (formerly the Sports Legacy Institute) was interviewed for *Popular Science* in 2012 and described the importance of rotational acceleration: "Because most hits are off-center and because our heads are not square, most of the accelerations in the head are going to be rotational" (Foster 2012). The exclusion of rotational force testing, up to and including current NOCSAE standards, represents a significant departure from current scientific knowledge about the mechanisms of concussive injuries.

Rotational hits are not modeled in current safety standards, and until recently were not modeled by Virginia Tech's STAR rating system. This remains the case despite the fact that the literature on helmet safety is quite consistent on this point (Lloyd and Conidi 2014; Sone et al. 2017). Lloyd and Conidi write, "While football helmets provide excellent protection from linear impacts—those leading to bruising and skull fracture—they offer little or no protection against rotational forces, a dangerous source of brain injury and encephalopathy" (2014). Collectively, these researchers warn their colleagues that current testing procedures systematically miss an important cause of brain injuries, including concussion.

Deficits in knowledge about the degree of protection helmets provide from the forces of rotational acceleration are clear to researchers and scientists in this field. Yet current safety standards, NOCSAE certification, and the Virginia Tech STAR ratings conceal this fact from consumers. Here we find an example of what Frickel calls "acknowledged ignorance" (Frickel 2014b). Researchers know that modeling rotational acceleration is difficult, and that contemporary practice does not measure it well. There is a disconnect between what is known about the biomechanics of concussion and how helmets are tested under the current NOCSAE certification. Frickel writes that sociologists of science and knowledge should investigate, "how the institutional structure of scientific fields produce and manage ignorance as a regular consequence of scientific business-as-usual" (Frickel 2014b, 270). Helmets were given a STAR rating and a NOCSAE seal. Both symbols promise maximal safety, yet obscure information about what was left out of the standards and testing protocols: what scientists have known from experimental studies about rotational force being the most likely mechanism of concussive injury (Duma and Rowson 2014). These facts might surprise the public and most consumers of football helmets. The veil of standards operates in this way: it conceals uncertainty and systematic gaps in commonly used metrics—metrics that themselves are subject to revision.

Updating NOCSAE Helmet Safety Standards

NOCSAE has responded to the growing calls for rotational acceleration tests with newly updated standards currently pending approval. Implementation, however, as previously noted, has been delayed from November 2018 to May 2019, and then again to November 2019. Without full access to NOCSAE records, it is difficult to understand why implementation is stalled. Perhaps technical issues with testing procedures have delayed implementation. Alternatively, it could be that manufacturer's internal testing has revealed inadequacies in their current testing models. We simply do not know.

As previously suggested, the new standards add a pneumatic ram impact test to assess safety but apply only to newly manufactured helmets. These guidelines, published as NOCSAE DOC (ND)002–17m19, specify that four samples of each helmet model should be tested, with two subject to the drop test and two subject to the pneumatic ram test. The pneumatic ram test uses compressed air to propel a 2.3 kg disc-shaped impactor head with a radius of about 127 mm into the helmet, which sits on a freely rotating neck assembly. The test assesses rotational force from impacts at six different locations on the helmet at velocities of 6 meters per second in adult helmets and 5.2 meters per second for youth helmets. From these tests, a "severity index" is calculated. The index is made up of a figure that represents the acceleration caused by drop or pneumatic ram impact expressed as the integration of acceleration over time in seconds over the duration of the acceleration pulse. NOCSAE considers helmets to have failed if their severity index rating is above 1,200 on any impact. In addition, the pending guidelines specify that any peak rotational acceleration of a medium headform on the pneumatic arm test above 6,000 radians per second squared also fails the test (NOCSAE DOC (ND)002–17m19). These standards may be considered an improvement in that they are responsive to concerns about rotational acceleration. Perhaps researchers will determine that new helmets do meet these standards, and public health researchers, ethicists, and others will be satisfied. I think this outcome is unlikely. This is, in part, because the revised standards still involve separate tests for linear and rotational forces. As noted above, nearly all real-world impacts involve both linear and rotational acceleration. Separating the tests, then, represents a departure from the conditions under which helmets are most often used.

Under current and pending standards, then, newly manufactured helmets are assessed for safety in ways that do not adequately replicate the conditions under which players use the equipment. At this time, it is difficult to know how common hard-shell helmets and newer, more pliable models such as VICIS Zero1 will test under the updated standards, although the Zero1 is currently a top-rated helmet in the Virginia Tech rankings. Newer models such as the Zero1 tend to be more expensive, with top-rated helmets according to NFL/NFLPA-sponsored tests costing nearly $1,000 each. Of the 16 helmets given five-star ratings under the Virginia Tech STAR system, four cost over $900, with the most expensive model, the Riddell Precision-FIT, priced at $1,700 (Rowson 2019). Nevertheless, if implemented as planned in November 2019, helmets tested under the new NOCSAE standards will carry the organization's official seal and be made available to in the U.S. Consumers will once again be subject to the veil of standards, as NOCSAE certification provides the appearance of scientific authority, while simultaneously misleading the public since testing procedures do not mimic real-world conditions. Players at the youth, college, and professional levels will continue to use equipment, potentially unaware that current standards may fail to protect them from concussions—hazards that are known but whose probability for any one player on any given play is uncertain. What is needed, following Stirling, is a robust process of social appraisal, consistent with the precautionary principle (2007).

Conclusion: Why Helmet Standards Matter

Football is a collision sport, characterized by repeated impacts to the body and brain for most every player. Organizations like the NCAA were founded, in part, as a response to skull fractures and deaths on the football field (Harrison 2014). NOCSAE was similarly organized out of concerns over deaths resulting from skull fracture. Fainaru-Wada and Fainaru's book (2013) documents that Dr. Elliott Pellman, then chair of the NFL's mild traumatic brain injury committee, was enthusiastic about creating a "super helmet" to prevent concussions. Neurosurgeon and concussion researcher Robert Cantu is reported to have considered the effort both "appealing and remarkably naïve," according to Fainaru-Wada and Fainaru (2013, 136). As noted in the introduction, such efforts are one example of a more general phenomenon where concern over mild traumatic brain injury are downplayed by league officials such as NFL commissioner Goodell (see Bachynski and Goldberg 2014 for an application to youth football and hockey). Unfortunately, no super helmet exists, although the NFL's Play Smart, Play Safe initiative recently awarded funding to two companies for products that hope to improve helmet performance (NFL Enterprises 2019). The program has awarded over $16M in grants since 2017 (NFL Enterprises 2019). Efforts to improve brain safety through changes to helmet padding and design continue despite evidence from biomechanical engineers and other experts. Fainaru-Wada and Fainaru (2013) report that Biokinetics, an Ottawa biomechanics firm, warned the helmet maker: "In a November 2000 confidential report to Riddell warning that no football helmet—no matter how new and improved—could prevent concussions" (184). Investigating the details of and changes in NOCSAE standards, and Virginia Tech's efforts to compare football helmets, we gain a better understanding of the state of helmet safety science, and the way in which standards operate to both reveal and conceal important information. This process, which I have called the veil of standards, reinforces inequality in the knowledge base of equipment makers, testers, and NOCSAE on one hand, and consumers and players on the other. The former groups have better access to knowledge on the strengths and deficits of existing standards and testing procedures in addition to active framing and shaping of future research. The latter group, in contrast, may be unaware of their epistemic disadvantage, as the challenges of assessing brain injury using existing standards is concealed.

This case points to the relevance of sociological theories of knowledge to understandings of collision and other contact sports. Frickel writes that researchers who wish to study ignorance should pay attention "to the rules that actors follow as they work around undone science" (Frickel 2014a, 93). In Frickel's case, federal and state officials generated health risk standards based on incomplete sampling procedures in addition to replacing the unknown risks of certain chemicals with the known risk of other, "comparable" chemicals whose risk profiles were known. When published and distributed through insurance agencies, public health authorities, and the public, the absence of knowledge regarding the toxicity of certain chemicals was erased. In the same way, knowledge about what helmet safety standards currently lack is obscured when helmets are given NOCSAE certification and sold in the market.

In the context of football helmet standards and ratings, researchers rely on testing protocols that have been used since the early 1970s despite research suggesting rotational impacts are more important to the etiology of concussion. Until the pending update, NOCSAE standards have not kept pace with growing recognition from researchers that rotational acceleration contributes more significantly to concussion than past studies previously acknowledged (Duma and Rowson 2014; Guskiewicz and Mihalik 2011; Kleiven 2013; Post and Hoshizaki 2015). Researchers such as Stefan Duma are currently developing a new equation that models effects of linear and rotational forces in helmeted impacts.

At present, NOCSAE's standards offer parents and public health officials a false sense of security. While it is certainly the case that no helmet can prevent concussions, it is also true that manufacturers such as Riddell have claimed that their helmets reduce the risk of concussion in youth with little to no evidentiary basis for that claim (Fainaru-Wada and Fainaru 2013). A recent class action lawsuit filed against Riddell and Easton Sports alleged that these companies advertised their helmets as more likely to prevent concussion than their competitors' products. When this case was decided, all claims against Easton-Bell Sports and six of eight claims against Riddell were dismissed by U.S. District Judge Paul Huck. Although Riddell had claimed its helmet would prevent concussions, Huck ruled that the helmet maker was not liable even though these claims were demonstrated to be untrue as players sustained these brain injuries (Packel 2012). Riddell's legal problems continue, with recent lawsuits filed in Texas (Caplan 2017) and Ohio (Kosman 2018).

The systematic lack of knowledge regarding rotational acceleration is one of the many gaps in our understanding of both the concussion crisis and the long-term effects of collision sports like football. Tellingly, *League of Denial* ends with an Afterword devoted to ongoing litigation and controversy over what the NFL knew and when. The last paragraph reads:

> Perhaps most telling was the research that wasn't being conducted. The one piece of information most relevant to football's future was the percentage of players expected to get brain damage. There were some ominous numbers out there (none more than [Boston University neuropathologist Anne] McKee's 59 out of 62). But McKee admitted her figures were skewed; all the players had been symptomatic before they died. She knew that nothing could be said definitively until players—healthy and diseased—could be tracked over the lengths of their careers and beyond.

The league knew this. The players knew this. The scientists knew this. And yet, as of this writing, there was no such study in the pipeline.

(Fainaru-Wada and Fainaru 2013, 361)

Starting in 2014, the NCAA and Department of Defense "CARE Consortium" is conducting a longitudinal study to track a cohort of about 40,000 student athletes and cadets (NCAA Sport Science Institute n.d.). Longitudinal studies like this allow researchers to compare participants' brain imaging at the start of the study to subsequent scans and relating any changes to head impact exposure. This group has published several papers concerning the effects of concussion, age of first concussion, and reliability of assessment tools for concussion. Only baseline data from NCAA athletes has been reported thus far (Katz et al. 2018). Organizations like the NCAA and NFL have extensive resources and the ability to sponsor important research like the CARE Consortium Study. Still, such efforts may be limited by inherent conflicts of interest. Research findings have the potential to undermine each organization's claim that football can be played in ways that minimize the risk to an acceptable level.

Perhaps the science will improve, resulting in more knowledge and non-knowledge produced, uncertainty reduced, and the game will continue. NOCSAE and Virginia Tech have each implemented new measures of rotational acceleration that is collected alongside linear acceleration data. These measures may give parents, coaches, and other stakeholders the information they need to assess the risk of concussion and long-term brain damage. What is still unclear, however, is the substantive effects of these new testing protocols and the downstream effects on helmet design. Future helmets will need to attain NOCSAE certification and will likely be tested using the STAR system; just how well they will perform remains an open question.

Stirling shows us how football players, public health advocates, leagues, coaches, and others should use the precautionary principle in situations characterized by ignorance, and contrasts this response with conditions in which risk analysis is more appropriate. He suggests that, in the face of uncertainty, ambiguity, or ignorance, policy decisions should be made by diverse stakeholders in a "social appraisal" process (2007, 313). Such processes would include individuals and stakeholder groups that have little or no conflicts of interest due to personal or corporate financial or reputational investments. Such procedures might examine a variety of scenarios, searching for gaps in knowledge and divergent perspectives, and admitting a full range of potential harms, and advocate early intervention and systemic analysis of potential harms (Stirling 2007).

Future research must deal with the practical issues of tracking an unfolding situation regarding the bodies and brains of youth, college, and adult football players. This calls for careful and pragmatic work uncovering the uncertainties, ambiguities, and other forms of knowledge and non-knowledge, that are created in this complex and dynamic field.

References

Bachynski, Kathleen E. 2016. "No Game for Boys to Play Debating the Safety of Youth Football, 1945–2015." Ph.D., Public Health, Columbia University, New York.

Bachynski, Kathleen E., and Daniel S. Goldberg. 2014. "Youth Sports & Public Health: Framing Risks of Mild Traumatic Brain Injury in American Football and Ice Hockey." *The Journal of Law, Medicine & Ethics* 42 (3): 323–333.

Bachynski, Kathleen E., and Daniel S. Goldberg. 2018. "Time Out: Nfl Conflicts of Interest with Public Health Efforts to Prevent Tbi." *Injury Prevention* 24 (3): 180–184.

Belson, Ken, and Benedict Carey. 2019. "Abnormal Levels of a Protein Linked to C.T.E. Found in N.F.L Players' Brains, Study Shows." *The New York Times*. New York: The New York Times Company.

Binney, Zachary O. and Kathleen E. Bachynski. 2019. "Estimating the Prevalence at Death of Cte Neuropathology among Professional Football Players." *Neurology* 92 (1): 43–45.

Borden, Sam. 2012. "Despite Risks, N.F.L. Leaves Helmet Choices in Players' Hands." *The New York Times*. New York: New York Times Company.

Caplan, Jeff. 2017. "Fort Worth Firm Files Concussion Lawsuit Against Helmet Maker Riddell." *Fort Worth Star-Telegram*, April 16, 2019. www.star-telegram.com/news/local/community/fort-worth/article129912509.html.

Chuck, Elizabeth. 2018. "Despite Evidence, Skeptics Try to Cast Doubt on Cte-Football Link." *NBC Universal*, August 30. www.nbcnews.com/news/sports/despite-evidence-skeptics-try-cast-doubt-cte-football-link-n897416.

Croissant, Jennifer L. 2014. "Agnotology: Ignorance and Absence or Towards a Sociology of Things That Aren't There." *Social Epistemology* 28 (1): 4–25. doi:10.1080/02691728.2013.862880.

Daniel, Ray W., Steven Rowson, and Stefan M. Duma. 2012. "Head Impact Exposure in Youth Football." *Annals of Biomedical Engineering* 40 (4): 976–981. doi:10.1007/s10439-012-0530-7.

Davidson, Kavitha A. 2015. "The Nfl Knocks out Its Concussion Study." *Bloomberg View* February 23. Web. January 12, 2016.

Duma, Stefan M., and Steven Rowson. 2014. "The Biomechanics of Concussion: 60 Years of Experimental Research." In *Concussions in Athletics: From Brain to Behavior*, edited by S.M. Slobounov, and W.J. Sebastianelli, 115–137. New York: Springer.

Fainaru-Wada, Mark, and Steve Fainaru. 2013. *League of Denial: The NFL, Concussions, and the Battle for Truth*. New York: Three Rivers Press.

Feudtner, Chris, and Steven H. Miles. 2018. "Traumatic Brain Injury News Reports and Participation in High School Tackle Football." *JAMA Pediatrics* 172 (5): 492–494.

Foster, Tom. 2012. "New Football Helmet Could Save the Sport." *Popular Science*, www.popsci.com/science/article/2013-08/helmet-wars-and-new-helmet-could-protect-us-all#page-15.

Frickel, Scott. 2014a. "Not Here and Everywhere: The Non-Production of Scientific Knowledge." In *Routledge Handbook of Science, Technology, and Society*, 263–276. London: Taylor & Francis

Frickel, Scott. 2014b. "Absences: Methodological Note About Nothing, in Particular." *Social Epistemology* 28 (1): 86–95. doi:10.1080/02691728.2013.862881.

Frickel, Scott, Sahra Gibbon, Jeff Howard, Joanna Kempner, Gwen Ottinger, and David J Hess. 2010. "Undone Science: Charting Social Movement and Civil Society Challenges to Research Agenda Setting." *Science, Technology, & Human Values* 35 (4): 444–473.

Fuhrmeister, Chris. 2014. "This May Be the Helmet That Solves Football's Concussion Crisis." *Business Insider*, May 30, 2019. www.businessinsider.com/helmet-football-concussion-2014-3.

Goffman, Erving. 1959. *The Presentation of Self in Everyday Life*. Garden City, NY: Doubleday Anchor.

Goldberg, Daniel S. 2013. "Mild Traumatic Brain Injury, the National Football League, and the Manufacture of Doubt: An Ethical, Legal, and Historical Analysis." *Journal of Legal Medicine* 34 (2): 157–191.

Guskiewicz, Kevin M., and Jason P. Mihalik. 2011. "Biomechanics of Sport Concussion: Quest for the Elusive Injury Threshold." *Exercise and Sport Sciences Reviews* 39 (1): 4–11.

Harrison, Emily A. 2014. "The First Concussion Crisis: Head Injury and Evidence in Early American Football." *American Journal of Public Health* 104 (5): 822–833. doi:10.2105/ajph.2013.301840.

Hess, David J. 2016. *Undone Science: Social Movements, Mobilized Publics, and Industrial Transitions*. Cambridge, MA: MIT Press.

Houck, Zachary, Breton Asken, Russell Bauer, Jason Pothast, Charlie Michaudet, and James Clugston. 2016. "Epidemiology of Sport-Related Concussion in an Ncaa Division I Football Bowl Subdivision Sample." *The American Journal of Sports Medicine* 44 (9): 2269–2275.

Institute, NCAA Sport Science. n.d. "Ncaa-Dod Care Consortium." *NCAA*, April 16, 2019. www.ncaa.org/sport-science-institute/topics/ncaa-dod-care-consortium.

Katz, Barry P., Maria Kudela, Jaroslaw Harezlak, Michael McCrea, Thomas McAllister, Steven P. Broglio, and CARE Consortium Investigators. 2018. "Baseline Performance of Ncaa Athletes on a Concussion Assessment Battery: A Report from the Care Consortium." *Sports Medicine* 48 (8): 1971–1985.

Kleiven, Svein. 2013. "Why Most Traumatic Brain Injuries Are Not Caused by Linear Acceleration but Skull Fractures Are." *Frontiers in Bioengineering and Biotechnology* 1 (15). doi:10.3389/fbioe.2013.00015.

Kosman, Josh. 2018. "Father Sues Football Helmet Makers Over Son's Cte-Related Death." *New York Post*, April 16, 2019. https://nypost.com/2018/05/31/father-sues-football-helmet-makers-over-sons-cte-related-death/.

Lawrence, David W., Michael G. Hutchison, and Paul Comper. 2015. "Descriptive Epidemiology of Musculoskeletal Injuries and Concussions in the National Football League, 2012–2014." *Orthopaedic Journal of Sports Medicine* 3 (5): 2325967115583653.

Lloyd, John, and Francis Conidi. 2014. "Comparison of Common Football Helmets in Preventing Concussion, Hemmorhage and Skull Fracture Using a Modified Drop Test." *Neurology* 82 (10 Supplement): P5.320.

Mariano, Willoughby, and Jennifer Peebles. 2017. "Tracking Concussions Can Help College Athletes, but Many Schools Don't." *The Atlanta Journal-Constitution*. Cox Media Group, December 28, 2017. www.ajc.com/news/tracking-concussions-can-help-college-athletes-but-many-schools-don/1zemNiMbVhHp6d2yahQUHP/.

McFarling, Usha Lee. 2019. "High-Tech Helmets Won't Solve the Nfl's Concussion Problem." *Los Angeles Times,* May 30, 2019. www.latimes.com/opinion/op-ed/la-oe-mcfarling-football-helmets-concussion-20190201-story.html.

McGoey, Linsey. 2012. "Strategic Unknowns: Towards a Sociology of Ignorance." *Economy and Society* 41 (1): 1–16.

National Research Council (NRC) and Institute of Medicine (IOM). 2014. *Sports-Related Concussions in Youth: Improving the Science, Changing the Culture.* Washington, DC: Institute of Medicine and National Research Council.

NFLPA. 2018. "NFL and Nflpa Release 2018 Helmet Laboratory Testing Performance Results." *NFL Players Association.* April 16, 2018. https://www.nflpa.com/news/2018-helmet-lab-testing-performance-results.

NFLPA. 2019. "NFL Announces Winners of Headhealthtech Challenge Vi." *NFL Enterprises,* June 3. www.playsmartplaysafe.com/newsroom/statements/nfl-announces-winners-headhealthtech-challenge-vi/

NOCSAE. n.d.-a. "Contact Nocsae." Overland Park, KS: National Operating Committee on Standards for Athletic Equipment, April 16, 2019. https://nocsae.org/about-nocsae/contact-nocsae/.

NOCSAE. n.d.-b. "History". April 16, 2019. https://nocsae.org/about-nocsae/history/.

NOCSAE. 2017. "Standard Test Method and Equipment Used in Evaluating the Performance Characteristics of Headgear/Equipment." P. 33, Vol. ND 001–17m17b. Overland Park, KS: National Operating Committee on Standards for Athletic Equipment.

NOCSAE. 2018a. *Football Helmet Standards Overview.* Edited by N. O. C. o. S. f. A. Equipment. Overland Park, KS: National Operating Committee on Standards for Athletic Equipment.

NOCSAE. 2018b. *Nocsae Overview.* Edited by N. O. C. o. S. f. A. Equipment. Overland Park, KS: NOCSAE.

NOCSAE. 2019a. January 8, 2019. https://nocsae.org/.

NOCSAE. 2019b. "Standard Performance Specification for Newly Manufactured Football Helmets." P. 7, Vol. (ND)002–17m19. Overland Park, KS: National Operating Committee on Standards for Athletic Equipment.

Packel, Dan. 2012, "Fla. Judge Knocks Down Football Helmet Concussion Suit." *Law360.com.* New York: Portfolio Media, Inc., January 9, 2019. www.law360.com/cases/4f3bb2f40a6ac714ec000004.

Papa, Linda, Semyon M. Slobounov, Hans C. Breiter, Alexa Walter, Tim Bream, Peter Seidenberg, Julian E. Bailes, Stephen Bravo, Brian Johnson, and David Kaufman, et al. 2018. "Elevations in Microrna Biomarkers in Serum Are Associated with Measures of Concussion, Neurocognitive Function, and Subconcussive Trauma over a Single National Collegiate Athletic Association Division I Season in Collegiate Football Players." *Journal of Neurotrauma* 36 (8): 1343–1351.

Post, Andrew, and T. Blaine Hoshizaki. 2015. "Rotational Acceleration, Brain Tissue Strain, and the Relationship to Concussion." *Journal of Biomechanical Engineering* 137 (3): 030801.

Rappert, Brian, and Wenda K. Bauchspies. 2014. "Introducing Absence." *Social Epistemology* 28 (1): 1–3. doi:02691728.2013.862875.

Rowson, Steven. 2019, "Virginia Tech Helmet Ratings." April 16. www.helmet.beam.vt.edu/varsity-football-helmet-ratings.html.

Rowson, Steven, and Stefan M. Duma. 2011. "Development of the Star Evaluation System for Football Helmets: Integrating Player Head Impact Exposure and Risk of Concussion." *Annals of Biomedical Engineering* 39 (8): 2130–2140. doi:10.1007/s10439-011-0322-5.

Solomon, Gary. 2018. "Chronic Traumatic Encephalopathy in Sports: A Historical and Narrative Review." *Developmental Neuropsychology*, 1–33.

Sone, Je Yeong, Douglas Kondziolka, Jason H. Huang, and Uzma Samadani. 2017. "Helmet Efficacy against Concussion and Traumatic Brain Injury: A Review." *Journal of Neurosurgery* 126 (3): 768–781.

Stirling, Andrew. 2007. "Risk, Precaution and Science: Towards a More Constructive Policy Debate: Talking Point on the Precautionary Principle." *EMBO Reports* 8 (4): 309–315.

Tagge, Chad A., Andrew M. Fisher, Olga V. Minaeva, Amanda Gaudreau-Balderrama, Juliet A. Moncaster, Xiao-Lei Zhang, Mark W. Wojnarowicz, Noel Casey, Haiyan Lu, Olga N. Kokiko-Cochran, Sudad Saman, Maria Ericsson, Kristen D. Onos, Ronel Veksler, Jr. Vladimir V. Senatorov, Asami Kondo, Xiao Z. Zhou, Omid Miry, Linnea R. Vose, Katisha R. Gopaul, Chirag Upreti, Christopher J. Nowinski, Robert C. Cantu, Victor E. Alvarez, Audrey M. Hildebrandt, Erich S. Franz, Janusz Konrad, James A. Hamilton, Ning Hua, Yorghos Tripodis, Andrew T. Anderson, Gareth R. Howell, Daniela Kaufer, Garth F. Hall, Kun P. Lu, Richard M. Ransohoff, Robin O. Cleveland, Neil W. Kowall, Thor D. Stein, Bruce T. Lamb, Bertrand R. Huber, William C. Moss, Alon Friedman, Patric K. Stanton, Ann C. McKee and Lee E. Goldstein. 2018. "Concussion, Microvascular Injury, and Early Tauopathy in Young Athletes after Impact Head Injury and an Impact Concussion Mouse Model." *Brain* 141 (2): 422–458. doi:10.1093/brain/awx350.

Taylor, Marshall A., Dustin S. Stoltz, and Terence E. McDonnell. 2019. "Binding Significance to Form: Cultural Objects, Neural Binding, and Cultural Change." *Poetics* 73: 1–16.

Vrentas, Jenny. 2018. "Tom Brady Can Keep His Old Helmet—for Now." *Sports Illustrated*, April 16, 2019.

Wallace, Matthew L., and Ismael Ràfols. 2018. "Institutional Shaping of Research Priorities: A Case Study on Avian Influenza." *Research Policy* 47 (10): 1975–1989.

5 What Does the Precautionary Principle Demand of Us? Ethics, Population Health Policy, and Sports-Related TBI

Daniel Goldberg

Introduction

The primary claim of this paper is that a robust understanding of the precautionary principle (PP) in population health carries significant ethical and policy implications regarding sports-related traumatic brain injury (TBI). Theoretical analysis of the PP has advanced in the last decade, and several recent monographs offer thoughtful frameworks both for understanding the ontology of the PP ("what is it?") and for its ethical significance in public health policy. This paper fleshes out a robust model for the PP, and then applies that framework to the maelstrom of issues swirling around sports-related TBI (especially those involving vulnerable groups such as children and youths). Despite the variety of perspectives on the precautionary principle, most commentators agree that the imperative to take a measured, and some might say *preventative*, approach is particularly relevant in cases where it is difficult to specify the extent of risk from a hazard to which large numbers of a vulnerable population are exposed. Sports-related TBI in children and youths is just such a case.

The PP, therefore, can shed light on crucial questions connected to TBI, including but not limited to:

1   What standards of evidence are needed to justify interventions designed to ameliorate the risk (understood in terms of both prevalence/incidence and severity)?
2   To what extent does the PP relax the standards of causality required to justify specific policy interventions?
3   Which (kinds of) interventions are justified based on imperfect evidence regarding the risks?

Application of a theoretically-robust framework for the PP in the context of sports-related TBI negates demands for strict standards of causality as a prerequisite for public health action. The PP is by its very definition a framework for making public health decisions without exact determinations of the specific causes or probabilities of relevant risks. It is crucial to thoroughly conceptualize the aims of the PP since calls to delay public health action in the absence of indisputable proof of causality have immense ethical and policy implications. Such demands have historically been deployed by regulated industry to downplay their association with health risks, a process commonly referred to as the "manufacture of doubt." This chapter argues that such demands related to establishing proof of causality have no place in policy discourse on sports-related TBI and should be rejected.

The Precautionary Principle: Concepts & Justifications

Although scholarly research on the theory and implications of the PP is not new, the last two decades have brought about an especially excellent body of work devoted to the subject (e.g., Steel 2015; Munthe 2011; Gardiner 2006; Weed 2004, 2010; Trouwborst 2002). This chapter expressly adopts Steel's perspective, for reasons that will become clear later in this chapter. At the outset, the questions considered in the current section are the most basic ones: What is the precautionary principle and why does it matter?

As virtually all discussions of the concept note, there are a variety of definitions for the PP. Steel's book begins with the observation that "the literature on PP is as a whole . . . disappointingly less than the sum of its parts. Although one finds many interesting insights and proposals related to PP, it is often unclear how these pieces fit together in a logically consistent manner" (Steel 2015, 12).[1] The principal error, according to Steel, is regarding the PP as either a "procedural requirement that constrains policymaking, a decision rule 'that aims to guide choices among specific . . . policies," or an epistemic rule 'that makes claims about how scientific inferences should proceed in light of risks of error'" (12). Rather, Steel posits that the PP embodies all three of these conceptions at once: it simultaneously serves as a protocol for the rigorous construction of public health policy, a method for deciding between potential courses of action, and a guide for determining how relevant scientific evidence should inform policy.

"Although Steel's argument that the PP is in part a decision rule and a procedural requirement is persuasive, I maintain that the epistemic rule is 'most important for ethical policymaking in population health'" (Goldberg 2016, 182). The epistemic dimension of the PP is most significant since it engages fundamental questions of policymaking: "What do we need to know in order to act? And what standards of evidence suffice to generate knowledge relevant to the decision for action?" (Goldberg 2016, 182). These questions demonstrate how the PP is relevant to requirements for public health action, which means that the PP is foundational to issues related to the assessment of knowledge and decision-making in public health. But how does the epistemic significance of the PP cash out in terms of specific policies and the arguments supporting them? The broader PP literature suggests that a form of epistemic crediting should be applied: the PP relaxes the standards of proof required to justify public health action.

What is at issue in the PP are questions of causation and the standards epistemic agents ought to require to morally justify public health action. Because such action is frequently, albeit not always, state action, such causal questions also have significant implications for robust processes of public reason and deliberative democracy, as well as for revealing the limits of public health law (Gostin and Wiley 2016). Steel points out that any adequate conceptual framework for the PP must provide specific guidance on the extent to which the boundaries of causal proof can be relaxed in the face of imperfect evidence. Steel articulates this point through what he calls the Meta-Precautionary Principle (MPP), which affirms that "uncertainty should not be a reason for inaction in the face of serious . . . threats" (2015, 21).[2] Arguments from the broader PP literature reinforce the logic of Steel's meta-precautionary principle and confirm that the PP demands a relaxation of the standards of proof required to justify public health action (Weed 2004; Munthe 2011).

The PP, moreover, is especially relevant in cases where it is difficult to specify the extent of risk from a hazard to which large numbers of a vulnerable population is exposed. This is exactly the epidemiologic situation that obtains with regard to youths and adolescents playing sports that appear to carry significant risks of TBI. Obviously, defining the scope of "significant" risks related to a specific activity is fraught not only for methodological reasons internal to the practice of injury surveillance, but also due to the immense social, political, and legal forces at work in the social imaginary surrounding games like tackle football in the U.S., ice hockey in Canada, and rugby or Australian-rules football in Australasia and parts of Europe.

Within these specific contexts, such sports are *deep play* (Goldberg 2008, 2013). Deep play games, according to Geertz (1972), are those that encode deep meaning for the society in which they are situated. Hence the extent to which risks of play are framed, managed, and ultimately tolerated (or not) reveals a tremendous amount about the values and interests of the respective societies in which actors enact deep play. Indeed, it is well-understood that different polities delineate the scope of the PP in very different ways and with different conceptions of what levels of risk tolerance justify policy intervention. Steel's model is useful because it provides a theoretical framework for determining how and when the PP justifies public health action, especially in relation to public health laws and policies. In the following section, I sketch out a fuller picture of the implications of Steel's model in the specific case of sports-related TBI.

The Precautionary Principle and Sport-Related TBI

It is important to delineate what is at stake in debates about sports-related TBI, especially in youths and adolescent sports contexts. Although, of course, there is substantial deliberation over how best to interpret the epidemiologic evidence connecting exposure to harm, there is also a crucial social and political question that is not simply a function of that empirical evidence base: to what risks is it acceptable to expose youths and adolescents? As Bachynski and I argued in 2014, this question is fundamentally normative in asking what we collectively ought to do. Answers to this question must, of course, be informed by the epidemiologic evidence, but that evidence base alone cannot *satisfy* the normative question. The question of what levels of risk are acceptable to expose youths and adolescents is a highly debatable one that will be resolved politically via (preferably robust) processes of public reason, or not at all.

In the U.S., tackle football is deep play. It is also the organized sport that presents some of the most significant risks of injury with long-term sequelae including but not limited to neuropathology. Unsurprisingly, then, public reason on the acceptability of the risks of sports-related TBI in the U.S. centers on tackle football. Therefore, while the scope of this paper addresses sports-related TBI in general, it is useful to pursue a specific deep play game—here, tackle football—to discern the impact of the PP in a specific social context. There is an increasingly vocal and persistent group of stakeholders in the U.S. arguing that, given the state of the evidence, it is ethically unacceptable to expose children and adolescents under the age of 14 to the risks of harm associated with tackle football (e.g., Nowinski and Cantu 2018; Frank 2018).[3] This argument is itself a call for an obvious policy intervention designed to ameliorate the harms associated with the relevant exposure (playing tackle football). Opponents of such an intervention have advanced multiple arguments against this claim, most of which center on the contention that the evidence of causation between exposure to tackle football and harms is insufficient to restrict or eliminate play for children under the age of 14 (Chung et al. 2018).

In my 2016 paper on demands for unreasonable proof of harm in debates over regulated industries accused of undermining population health, I identified an argument that has been repeatedly deployed by opponents of interventions that are designed to obstruct, curtail, or eliminate the particular product being marketed and sold. I called this logic, standardized argument *S*. A close analogue of standardized argument *S* is easily observable through the actions of opponents of interventions designed to obstruct, curtail, or eliminate U.S. tackle football for youths under the age of 14. Here is the form of the standardized argument *S* as it appears in policy and ethical discourse regarding sports-related TBI:

p_1: To justify policy obstructing, curtailing, or eliminating participation in tackle football for youth under the age of 14, harm to participants caused by such play must be shown.

p_2: Harm to play can only be shown by evidence of clinically meaningful outcomes.

p_3: Evidence of clinically meaningful outcomes requires proof of causation linking exposure and outcome.

p_4: Proof of causation linking exposure and outcome can only be generated via a double-blind, placebo-controlled, randomized controlled trial (RCT).

p_5:   Proof of causation linking exposure and outcome acquired via a double-blind, placebo-controlled, RCT has not been obtained in the context of participation in tackle football under the age of 14.

C: There is no justification for policies obstructing, curtailing, or eliminating participation in tackle football for participants under the age of 14.

To see how this argument pans out, note the contrapositive of p_1, in which the hypothesis and conclusion of the statement are reversed: If no harm to [players] caused by participation in tackle football for those under the age of 14 can be shown, "then the policy justification for curtailing or eliminating" such play "is substantially weakened. The . . . standard harm-based argument therefore centers on the criteria for proving harm" (Goldberg 2016, 178).

p^4 can be dispensed relatively quickly, since there is essentially a consensus rejecting the claim that proof of a causal exposure–harm link can only be shown via a randomized controlled trial (Goldberg 2016). Vigorous and repeated critiques have derailed the claim that RCTs represent some sort of mystical "gold standard" that always and forever sits atop an evidence hierarchy for any given epidemiologic question (Greenhalgh et al. 2014; LaCaze 2008; Grossman and Mackenzie 2005). Moreover, as I argued in my 2016 paper,

> even if we granted that RCTs are categorically the best evidence of a causal exposure–outcome link, there are immense obstacles to their implementation. First, RCTs are notoriously expensive. Second, when the outcome in question is connected to noncommunicable diseases . . . clinically meaningful outcomes may take years or even decades to measure, which substantially increases the risk of loss to follow-up, erosion of needed funds, etc. But above all, especially in the context of epidemiologic studies, RCTs may be indisputably unethical because they would require exposing the participants in the experimental arm to a known health hazard. . . . Hence, it is axiomatic that RCTs are often simply impossible to perform in epidemiologic research, whether for reasons of money, time, and/or ethics.
>
> (Goldberg 2016, 180)

p^3 is where the argument for the PP is especially significant, however, and will be the focal point of the remaining analysis. In the absence of ideal evidence for causal links between exposure-harm, what is to be done? Actually, for opponents of policies limiting or eliminating the exposure in question (participation in tackle football), the answer lies within the question itself: little to nothing. Perhaps this is an overstatement. Proponents of permitting youths and adolescents to repeatedly run into each other at top speed for years do come armed with proposals for "making the game safer." But given that there is little quality evidence suggesting that any interventions short of actual cessation of play can prevent harms associated with such play (Bachynski and

Goldberg 2014), the fighting issue in terms of risk reduction is whether play should be eliminated, at least for children and adolescents under the age of 14. Thus, for opponents of policies that seek to eliminate or severely restrict <14 participation in football, preservation of the status quo is the key policy message. Before proceeding to analysis of how and why the PP impacts the legitimacy of this argument, it is worth pausing to note the lengthy history of such efforts to preserve the status quo on the basis of perceived insufficient causal evidence of a given exposure-harm link.

History, the PP, and the Manufacture of Doubt

I have argued extensively that it is impossible to understand the debate over the issue of youth and adolescent participation in sports that pose substantial TBI risks outside of its historical and political context (Goldberg 2013; Bachynski and Goldberg 2014, 2018). Specifically, regulated industries accused of selling products causing population health harms have, for at least a century in the U.S., followed a historical script. This script is not a causal *deus ex machina*, but is rather the discursive product of a distinct social, political, and legal strategy designed primarily to forestall regulatory intervention. Its social power is why this strategy continues to be wielded by contemporaneous industry actors, including, of course, professional sports leagues connected to American football, ice hockey, and rugby, among others.

Developing around a deep and interdisciplinary literature drawing on tools from, inter alia, history, ethics, law, policy and decision sciences, epidemiology, and philosophy, the script has come to be termed "the manufacture of doubt." The phrase takes on its most evocative usage in the words of a high-ranking tobacco executive's internal memoranda reading, simply, "Doubt is our product" (Michaels 2008). Although historically, industry actors have utilized a wide variety of approaches to manufacture doubt about the harms of their products, several points stand out as significant strategies. First, industry actors have repeatedly asserted that causal evidence of an exposure-harm link was insufficient to require a stay on regulatory interventions. Second, the manufacture of doubt is associated with the phenomenon of regulatory capture, whereby regulatory bodies foreground the interests of the entities they are charged with regulating (rather than, e.g., public health, environmental safety, etc.). Administrative law essentially requires close contact between regulatory bodies and the industries being regulated. While there are advantages for such relationships for policy and practice, extensive evidence shows that deep relationships have a powerful effect on human behavior through the mechanism of motivated bias (for a discussion of this evidence, see Goldberg 2016). This means that the well-documented conflicts of interests with which regulatory bodies and officials grapple significantly shape the processes through which regulations and policies are carried out.

Third, since public opinion of regulated industries can turn decidedly negative, industry actors have repeatedly found it necessary to purchase social credibility. They cannot acquire it on their own, so they must form certain relationships with social actors who enjoy public acclaim and respect. Because concerns over population health are inherent to the manufacture of doubt—these regulated industries are at issue precisely because their products pose health hazards—the credibility of health professionals including public health scientists and expert clinicians are especially important to appropriate and mobilize for service in the manufacture of doubt. Medical historian Dominique Tobbell (2009, 2011) has traced this process expressly as it related to the nascent American pharmaceutical industry and physicians in the post-WWII era. It has also been well-documented in a variety of twentieth and twenty-first century regulated industries, including but not limited to vinyl, lead, asbestos, food, and, of course, tobacco.[4]

Although the manufacture of doubt supports a variety of social and political objectives, one of the most historically primary goals is to create what is known as a regulatory vacuum where, by definition, there is substantially less oversight. The first strategy, challenging the sufficiency of causal links between exposure and harm, has historically been especially significant in sustaining such a vacuum.

In turn, regulatory vacuums can induce serious population health effects; the most obvious example is the case of tobacco, as noted by David Michaels (2008): delays in regulation of tobacco products resulted in excess deaths in the thousands, if not the millions—not to mention dramatically elevated rates of illness and disease as well.[5] Yet there is similarly good evidence that both the U.S. National Football League and the National Hockey League have relied on each of these strategies in countering calls for policy-based interventions regarding sports-related TBI (Joyce 2018; Bachynski and Goldberg 2018). Numerous observers, including U.S. congressional legislators, have expressly noted the similarities between tobacco industry tactics and that deployed by the NFL (Paolini 2018; Goldberg 2013). In 2009 hearings before the U.S. Congress, Rep. Linda Sánchez (D-CA) stated that the NFL's denials "sort of reminds me of the tobacco companies pre-1990s when they kept saying 'No, there is no link between smoking and damage to your health or ill health effects'" (Legal Issues 2009, 116). Accordingly, one essential conclusion to draw from the historical evidence is that when opponents of <14 limitations on tackle football cite perceived insufficiency of the evidence of causation, they are both reflecting and extending older historical patterns of thought and action foundational to the manufacture of doubt. Even when claims of insufficient evidence are not directly intended to fuel the manufacture of doubt, deeply rooted historical scripts can have powerful social effects—and this is true even where the actor does not intend any such effects. The real power of historical scripts is not reducible to the intentions of the actors. Successful arguments that reify the manufacture of doubt, even unintentionally, can create and/or sustain regulatory and policy vacuums that might otherwise produce interventions intended to—and often with the capability to—reduce the risk of a harm associated with relevant exposures.

Finally, there is also an important conceptual connection between the manufacture of doubt and the precautionary principle. Steel argues that examining historical contexts is essential for demonstrating how rarely regulatory action on the basis of the PP has resulted in social harm:

> [E]nvironmental and public health history does not support the contention that the epistemic line justifying public health action has frequently been applied too loosely (and hence that precautions have been "excessive"). Rather, twentieth century environmental and public health history shows time and again examples where a regulated industry's successful manufacture of doubt created a regulatory vacuum that in retrospect caused immense harm.
>
> (Goldberg 2016, 184, citing Steel 2015, 69–94)

Given this juxtaposition, it is now possible to examine the implications of the PP for sports-related TBI, using the case of eliminating, curtailing, or severely restricting participation in American tackle football for children under the age of 14.

The Case of Tackle Football in Children & Adolescents Under the Age of 14

Playing American tackle football poses a risk of both neuropathology with potentially lifelong and life-limiting sequelae, as well as other comorbidities such as chronic pain and inflammatory disease (Evans 2017; Findler 2015; Domb et al. 2014; Golightly et al. 2011). As I mentioned earlier in this chapter, however, perhaps the most pressing question concerns the acceptable levels of risk to which to expose vulnerable groups like children and adolescents (Bachynski and Goldberg 2014). Again, this question cannot be answered solely from epidemiologic evidence clarifying degrees of risk, yet greater specification of the risk is nevertheless immensely helpful to informing the ethical inquiry itself. That is, we can sharpen the ethical debate around sports-related TBI by understanding the intricacies of the epidemiologic and empirical evidence.

Science connected to sports-related TBI is a relatively young field, although there are vigorous efforts underway to better understand, analyze, predict, treat, and prevent the risks associated with youth and adolescent participation in American tackle football. A variety of important questions remain unanswered, including, e.g., explanations for gender differences in prevalence and incidence, age-based differences, and the connections between sub-concussive injury and short-term vs. long-term neuropathology (Carman et al. 2015). Given the absence of irrefutable epidemiologic evidence enabling exact calibration of potential risks, then, what is the optimal policy intervention? What should be done? Again, there is little dispute over efforts to reduce TBI risk by making incremental changes to the game such as additional education and training, changing tackling techniques and penalizing or banning certain forms of play deemed especially dangerous. With one notable exception—banning body checking in youth ice hockey (Emery and Black 2019)—there is little evidence that such incremental changes have a substantial risk-reducing effect. Indeed, while Emery and Black note the evidence showing that eliminating this technique in ice hockey may substantially reduce incidence of all injuries, they also concede that further research is needed to justify any claim that rule changes in US football, rugby, lacrosse, or soccer can substantially reduce rates of injury. If there is little evidence that any intervention short of total cessation/prevention has much impact in reducing the inherent risks of sports such as tackle football and ice hockey, then the fighting issue is whether a policy intervention that calls for the elimination of participation in full-contact sports deemed especially dangerous under a given age is warranted.

The debate over this question has been playing out in real time for much of 2017 and 2018. At the time of this writing, five states had introduced legislation proposing a ban on >14 participation in tackle football: California, Illinois, Maryland, New Jersey, and New York. The arguments in favor of such a policy are supported by significant correlative and associative epidemiologic evidence regarding the psychological, orthopedic, and neurological health risks of participation in tackle football over the lifespan, most of which has been ably summarized elsewhere (Evans 2017; Findler 2015; Domb et al. 2014; Golightly et al. 2011). While none of these bills were enacted during 2017–18 legislative sessions, each effort was met with substantial media coverage and criticism. As an April 2018 feature in the *Orange County Register* explained,

> In each [state], the backlash was swift and unyielding. Coaches and parents flooded phone lines, email boxes and talk radio, condemning the bills and questioning the science behind them. Within weeks, three of five bills were dead or left in legislative purgatory, crushed under the weight of youth football's influence.
>
> (Karte 2018)

Again, consistent with the historical sweep of the manufacture of doubt (Goldberg 2016), opponents of these policies couched their position in terms of freedom and antagonism to government overreach (e.g., Karte 2018; Tim 2018). Critics also maintained that the evidence was insufficient to justify the interventions proposed (Sadin 2018; Fainaru-Wada and Steele 2018). These arguments tend to imitate, almost perfectly, the contentions wielded by generations of actors in service of the manufacture of doubt: there is insufficient evidence of a causal link between the exposure (play) and the harms (neuropathology).[6]

It is within such debates that the PP has particular relevance. The PP essentially relaxes the epistemic requirements for justification of public health action. The PP's epistemic implications are focused on the question of causal links between a given exposure and observed harms. As Steel and others, including myself, have noted, this relaxation is justifiable on a number of levels, not least because its absence essentially neuters public health action. For a variety of reasons, compelling proof of causation between a given exposure and harms is frequently lacking in public health contexts. For example, in population health contexts, it is frequently impossible to control for the large number of confounders to isolate the causal effects of a given exposure. In addition, as noted above, it is often unethical to conduct randomized controlled trials that can in some circumstances provide solid proof of causality: "We cannot, for example, conduct a RCT to discern the precise amount of lead exposure that destroys a child's liver function because the known harms of exposing child research subjects to lead's toxic effects vastly outweigh the good of determining more precise levels of toxicity" (Goldberg 2016, 180). Similarly, in a tackle football context, it would be patently unethical to intentionally expose children to increasing levels of force to determine the precise levels at which permanent brain damage will follow.

The PP, therefore, is a primary epistemic tool that justifies public health action in the face of imperfect evidence of causal links between specific exposures and population health harms. Of course, the rub is in the details; as virtually all PP scholars note, it cannot be a blank check justifying any and all public health action irrespective of deficiencies in the epidemiologic evidence connected to a specific exposure. There are, and must be, limits to the social spaces and contexts in which public health actions are justified, in no small part because the vast majority of such actions restrict various liberties and freedoms. For example, part of the vigorous objection to New York City Mayor Bloomberg's efforts to ban the sale of soda cups larger than 16 ounces was that the regulation represented a substantial restriction on freedom with very little evidence that doing so would improve population health (Studdert et al. 2015).

But these difficulties, while real, do not exist at the margins. That is, the intricate problems that exist in delineating the limits of the PP are not justification for dispensing with the PP entirely. Doing so essentially vitiates one of the primary epistemic justifications for public health action and would therefore result in disastrous public health consequences. Moreover, epidemiologists, public health professionals, and policymakers are hardly unaware of or inexperienced in dealing with the problems of causation so frequently encountered in public health contexts. Epidemiologists have developed a variety of methods for inferring causal relationships (multilevel modeling, the Bradford-Hill characteristics, etc.) There is widespread, albeit not uniform agreement among epidemiologists and decision scientists that, in assessing specific exposure-harm links, as more of the relevant evidentiary standards are satisfied, the better the justification for inferring causation and intervening (Vandenbroucke et al. 2016).

The argument here is simply that in assessing whether public health action is justified regarding a specific exposure-harm link, wielding the claim of "lack of causality" does not end the inquiry. The argument opposing public health action proves too much. If the lack of robust evidence of causation were adjudged sufficient to negate the justification for public health action, we would enjoy little, if any, public health action. "This consequence is absurd. The very real problems involved in determining the limits of justified public health action do not license the conclusion that public health action is ipso facto unjustifiable." (Goldberg 2016, 184). I trust that it needs little analysis to understand why essentially canceling public health action outright would be morally impermissible. Therefore, the PP has important moral content in thinking about public health ethics, or what Wikler and Brock (2007) termed "population-level bioethics." Demanding unreasonable standards for proof of harm in public health contexts also ignores standards for epidemiologic harm that are *generally accepted* within the relevant epistemic communities (i.e., epidemiologists and public health scientists). As I wrote in 2016, "Although problems of evidence and proof are of course significant within the practice of public health, epidemiologic science is unquestionably accepted by participants in that epistemic community as a legitimate basis for inferring causation to a level sufficient to merit public health action" (Goldberg 2016, 185).

Furthermore, opponents of the <14 bans have not specified what quantum of evidence would satisfy their strict demands for proof of causation. This too is consistent with the historical and political role of the strategy in the manufacture of doubt. Since it is ethically and practically impossible to run a RCT intended to assess the level at which the exposure of tackle football to children and adolescents produces the harm of long-term neuropathology, those who deny the sufficiency of the current state of the evidence should offer a precise delineation of the standards they deem necessary to justify policy interventions such as the <14 restriction. This is especially important given the history of the manufacture of doubt in the context of American football, through which claims of insufficient causal evidence have been used time and again to forestall *any* policy action and maintain the status quo (Goldberg 2013).

Finkel and Bieniek (2019) recently adopted a similar analysis in quantitating the risk of CTE in professional tackle football players. Tracking the U.S. Occupational Health & Safety Administration's general approach to quantitative risk assessments, Finkel and Bieniek estimate the "lowest possible risk estimates" for a cohort of 17,150 player-careers over the last 45 years from "6.4 per thousand to . . . 13 per thousand" (17). These figures are estimates of the rusk that a professional tackle football player will develop chronic traumatic encephalopathy. They observe that these estimates are biased towards the null, which means that *whatever* the actual risk is very likely exceeds the risk-estimate range they offer. Biasing towards the null is a technique often used in epidemiology to assess risk, since it means that scientists need not be able to specify the actual risk: where all assumptions and parameters are biased towards zero, the actual risk is almost certainly greater than the range offered in the estimation. Finkel and Bieniek (2019) also note that the risk-estimates easily exceed the levels of quantitated risk at which OSHA typically initiates regulatory, preventive, and protective action. They conclude that scientific regulatory communities in the US have historically and consistently used generally accepted risk and evidence paradigms in implementing policy and precautions intended to protect population health.

Ultimately, demands for strict standards of causality as a prerequisite for public health action are generally unjustified and should be rejected. The PP serves to relax the epistemic standards of proof required to justify public health and policy intervention. Although rigorous epidemiologic evidence of causal links between play and health harms would be ideal, the PP gives justification for action in preventing potentially significant harm to a vulnerable population in the absence of that evidence. This is the point of the PP, and the legacy of public health history makes quite clear that the consequences of ignoring the epistemic and evidentiary warrant provided by the PP can be devastating (Steel 2015). By urging a preservation of the status quo, opponents of calls to ban or severely limit participation in inherently dangerous sports like football, ice hockey, rugby, or boxing are essentially gutting the PP. As noted earlier, if public health actions generally required the kinds of evidence that opponents of such policies tend to demand, there would essentially be no public health action at all. This is an absurd consequence. Such a demand has no justifiable place in policy discourse on sports-related TBI and should be rejected.

Conclusion

Under the capacious epistemic warrant provided by the PP, there is ample epidemiologic evidence from which to justify policies that ban or severely limit <14 participation in sports that pose significant risks of TBI and other life-altering morbidities. The PP demonstrates why not knowing the precise level of risk at the present time is a poor justification for arguing for the status quo is preferable policy.

That being said, it is certainly possible to argue against calls to ban or severely limit <14 tackle football for reasons beyond insufficient proof of causality. For example, one might claim that the benefits of <14 participation outweigh potential risks of harm, and that an outright ban might deprive youths from important experiences and life lessons. However dubious such arguments may be, the important point is that these claims do not suffer from the infirmities of the arguments based on insufficiency of evidence of causation. The latter are rooted in profoundly troubling and historically harmful scripts that have been consciously and repeatedly deployed by powerful industry actors and their allies to forestall regulatory action and preserve the status quo. Such arguments proceed either in ignorance or contravention of the PP, and demand unreasonable standards for proof of harm that are rejected by the most relevant epistemic communities (epidemiologists and public health scientists).

Ultimately, the decision on whether and when it is appropriate for youths and adolescents to participate in sports—or activities in general—that pose significant risks of TBI is a complex moral, social, and political inquiry. Reasonable people of good conscience can and do disagree on the acceptability of exposing children to risks the precise measures of which are largely unknown. But robust processes of deliberative democracy (Gutmann and Thompson 2009) and public reason needed to resolve the problem should not include the types of arguments urging preservation of the status quo on the basis of insufficient proof of causation. Such arguments are specious, contravene the epistemic and ethical warrant of the PP, and have contributed to immense and inequitably distributed population health harms for over a century. Such arguments should be rejected wherever they appear, and preferably absented from public and policy discourse entirely.

Notes

1. This summary and discussion of Steel's framework flows in large part from a prior use to which I put it (Goldberg 2016). That prior effort, addressing conflicts of interest and justifiable standards of causality, is relevant to this paper, and will be discussed in Section III.
2. The meta-precautionary principle is one of what Steel identifies as three core components of the PP. The MPP enjoys the other two components, the "tripod" and a proportionality component. The tripod itself consists of (1) a knowledge condition; (2) a harm condition; and (3) a recommended precaution. Steel's model is complex and full explication of the tripod is neither germane nor especially helpful here.
3. The justification for drawing the line at 14 years of age for participation in tackle football is complex and is essentially beyond the scope of this paper. While there is evidence that neck muscles are more developed by this age and therefore that players may be better able to protect themselves, neurodevelopment continues in earnest until the early 20s. More importantly, there is little evidence showing the quantum of the risk reduction that results in permitting play at age 14 vs. ages 7–13. Nor is there evidence documenting how much risk could further be reduced by barring play until adolescents are older (say, 15–18). Nevertheless, the policy arguments in the US are currently squarely centered on the 14-year-old-boundary, and this is therefore the subject of analysis in this section.
4. In general, the large body of work produced by historians Allan Brandt, David Rosner, Gerald Markowitz, and Gerald Oppenheimer ground these claims.
5. This example is also a plain demonstration of the idea that law and policy is a major social determinant of health in its own right, an observation that is core to the developing fields of public health law research and legal epidemiology.
6. A serious omission in this analysis is the fact that virtually no opponent of calls to limit or ban <14 participation in full-contact sports addresses the risks of any health harm *other than* neuropathology. This is a significant flaw, because the causal links between play and other morbidities—most notably chronic pain and inflammatory disease—are much better established and are not currently in serious dispute. Given the immense social costs of these noncommunicable diseases, omitting them from the risk-benefit analysis is a morally and politically unacceptable oversight. I hope to address this point in future work.

References

Bachynski, Kathleen E., and Daniel S. Goldberg. 2014. "Youth Sports & Public Health: Framing Risks of Mild Traumatic Brain Injury in American Football and Ice Hockey." *The Journal of Law, Medicine & Ethics* 42 (3): 323–333.

Bachynski, Kathleen E., and Daniel S. Goldberg. 2018. "Time Out: NFL Conflicts of Interest with Public Health Efforts to Prevent TBI." *Injury Prevention* 24 (3): 180–184.

Carman, Aaron J., Rennie Ferguson, Robert Cantu, R. Dawn Comstock, Penny A. Dacks, Steven T. DeKosky, Sam Gandy, et al. 2015. "Mind the Gaps-advancing Research into Short-Term and Long-term Neuropsychological Outcomes of Youth Sports-related Concussions." *Nature Reviews Neurology* 11 (4): 230–245.

Chung, J., P. Cummings, and U. Samadani. 2018. Does CTE call for an End to Youth Tackle Football? *The Minneapolis Star-Tribune.* http://www.startribune.com/does-cte-call-for-an-end-to-youth-tackle-football/473655913/

Domb, Benjamin G., Chris Carter, Nathan A. Finch, Jon E. Hammarstedt, Kevin F. Dunne, and Christine E. Stake. 2014. "Whole-person Impairment in Younger Retired NFL Players: The Orthopaedic Toll of a Professional Football Career." *Orthopaedic Journal of Sports Medicine* 2 (5): 2325967114534824.

Emery, Carolyn A., and Amanda M. Black. 2019. "Are Rule Changes the Low-hanging Fruit for Concussion Prevention in Youth Sport?" *JAMA Pediatrics* 2019173 (4): 309–310.

Evans, Randolph W. 2017. "The Prevalence of Migraine and Other Neurological Conditions Among Retired National Football League Players: A Pilot Study." *Practical Neurology*, November/December 21–25.

Fainaru-Wada, M., and M. Steele. 2018. "Debate Over Youth Tackle Football an Extension of Country's Polarized Politics." *ESPN*, September 27. www.espn.com/espn/otl/story/_/id/24773919/efforts-ban-youth-tackle-football-five-states-draw-comparisons-nanny-state-grass-roots-politics

Findler, Patrick. 2015. "Should Kids Play (American) Football?" *Journal of the Philosophy of Sport* 42 (3): 443–462.

Finkel, Adam M., and Kevin F. Bieniek. 2019. "A Quantitative Risk Assessment for Chronic Traumatic Encephalopathy (CTE) in Football: How Public Health Science Evaluates Evidence." *Human and Ecological Risk Assessment: An International Journal* 25 (3): 564–589.

Frank, Noah. 2018. "Maryland to Introduce Bill to Ban Tackle Football Under Age 14." *WTOP*, February 5. https://wtop.com/maryland/2018/02/maryland-to-introduce-bill-to-ban-tackle-football-under-age-14/

Gardiner, Stephen M. 2006. "A Core Precautionary Principle." *Journal of Political Philosophy* 14 (1): 33–60.

Geertz, Clifford. 1972. "Deep Play: Notes on the Balinese Cockfight." *Daedalus* 101 (1): 1–37.

Goldberg, Daniel S. 2008. "Concussions, Professional Sports, and Conflicts of Interest: Why the National Football League's Current Policies are Bad for Its (Players') Health." *HEC Forum* 20 (4): 337–355.

Goldberg, Daniel S. 2013. "Mild Traumatic Brain Injury, the National Football League, and the Manufacture of Doubt: An Ethical, Legal, and Historical Analysis." *Journal of Legal Medicine* 34 (2): 157–191.

Goldberg, Daniel S. 2016. "On Physician—Industry Relationships and Unreasonable Standards of Proof for Harm: A Population-Level Bioethics Approach." *Kennedy Institute of Ethics Journal* 26 (2): 173–194.

Golightly, Yvonne M., Stephen W. Marshall, and Dennis J. Caine. 2011. "Future Shock: Youth Sports and Osteoarthritis Risk." *Lower Extremity Review*, October.

Gostin, Lawrence O., and Lindsay F. Wiley. 2016. *Public Health Law: Power, Duty, Restraint*. Oakland, CA: University of California Press.

Greenhalgh, Trisha, Jeremy Howick, and Neal Maskrey. 2014. "Evidence Based Medicine: A Movement in Crisis?" *BMJ* 348: g3725.

Grossman, Jason. 2008. "A Couple of the Nasties Lurking in Evidence-Based Medicine." *Social Epistemology* 22 (4): 333–352.

Grossman, J. and Mackenzie, F.J., 2005. The randomized controlled trial: gold standard, or merely standard?. *Perspectives in biology and medicine* 48 (4), pp. 516–534.

Gutmann, Amy, and Dennis Thompson. 2009. *Why Deliberative Democracy?* Princeton, NJ: Princeton University Press.

Joyce, M. Is the NFL using the CDC to 'manufacture doubt' on head injuries? Retrieved from https://www.healthnewsreview.org/2018/01/nfl-cdc-tbi162490/.

Karte, Ryan. 2018. "Law to Ban Tackle Football for California Youth Falls Short of Committee." *Orange County Register*, April 27. www.ocregister.com/2018/04/27/law-to-ban-tackle-football-for-california-youth-falls-short-of-committee/.

La Caze, Adam. 2008. "Evidence-based Medicine Can't Be . . ." *Social Epistemology* 22 (4): 353–370.

Legal Issues Relating to Football Head Injuries. 2009. "(Part I & II): Hearing Before the Committee on the Judiciary House of Representatives." *111th Cong*, 138. www.govinfo.gov/content/pkg/CHRG-111hhrg53092/html/CHRG-111hhrg53092.htm

Michaels, David. 2008. *Doubt Is Their Product: How Industry's Assault on Science Threatens Your Health*. Oxford: Oxford University Press.

Munthe, Christian. 2011. *The Price of Precaution and the Ethics of Risk* (Vol. 6). New York: Springer Science & Business Media.

Nowinski, C.J., and Robert Cantu. 2018. *Flag Football under 14: An Education Campaign for Parents*. Concussion Legacy Foundation. https://concussion foundation.org/sites/default/files/Documents/Flag_Under_14_White_Paper.pdf

Paolini, Mikayla. 2018. "NFL Takes a Page from the Big Tobacco Playbook: Assumption of Risk in the CTE Crisis." *Emory Law Journal* 68: 607.

Sadin, Steve. 2018. "Bill That Would Ban Tackle Football for Kids Under 12 in Illinois Won't Be Called for Vote, Likely Is Dead." *Chicago Tribune*, April 18. www.chicagotribune.com/news/breaking/ct-met-tackle-football-ban-bill-illinois-20180418-story.html.

Shen, Francis X. 2018. "You Can Love the Brain and Football, Too." *Minneapolis Star-Tribune*, January 31. www.startribune.com/youth-football-and-concussions-i-love-the-brain-but-think-you-can-like-football-too/472033803/

Steel, Daniel. 2015. *Philosophy and the Precautionary Principle*. Cambridge, UK: Cambridge University Press.

Studdert, David M., Jordan Flanders, and Michelle M. Mello. 2015. "Searching for Public Health Law's Sweet Spot: The Regulation of Sugar-sweetened Beverages." *PLoS Medicine* 12 (7): e1001848.

Tim, Edgy. 2018. "Should Under-12 Tackle Football be Banned in Illinois?" *NBC Sports*, March 2. www.nbcsports.com/chicago/preps-talk/should-under-12-tackle-football-be-banned-illinois.

Tobbell, Dominique A. 2009. "'Who's Winning the Human Race?' Cold War as Pharmaceutical Political Strategy." *Journal of the History of Medicine and Allied Sciences* 64 (4): 429–473.

Tobbell, Dominique A. 2011. *Pills, Power, and Policy: The Struggle for Drug Reform in Cold War America and Its Consequences* (Vol. 23). Oakland, CA: University of California Press.

Trouwborst, Adam. 2002. *Evolution and Status of the Precautionary Principle in International Law.* New York: Springer.

Vandenbroucke, Jan P., Alex Broadbent, and Neil Pearce. 2016. "Causality and Causal Inference in Epidemiology: The Need for a Pluralistic Approach." *International Journal of Epidemiology* 45 (6): 1776–1786.

Weed, Douglas L. 2004. "Precaution, Prevention, and Public Health Ethics." *The Journal of Medicine and Philosophy* 29 (3): 313–332.

Weed, D. L. (2010). Meta-analysis and causal inference: a case study of benzene and non-Hodgkin lymphoma. *Annals of epidemiology* 20 (5): 347–355.

Wikler, Daniel, and Dan W. Brock. 2007. "Population-level Bioethics: Mapping a New Agenda." *Ethics, Prevention, and Public Health,* 78–94.

Part III

The Politics of Trauma, Experience, and Research

6 "I Kinda' Lost My Sense of Who I Was"

Foregrounding Youths' Experiences in Critical Conversations About Sport-Related Concussions

William Bridel, Matt Ventresca, Danika Kelly, Kevin Viliunas, and Kathryn Schneider

As sport-related concussion has become a topic of significant cultural concern over the past decade, academics have both responded and contributed to this growth in public interest. The increasing scholarly focus on sport-related concussion has emerged most strikingly within the medico-scientific fields of neuroscience, medicine, rehabilitation, neuropsychology, and epidemiology. Socio-cultural researchers have also entered—perhaps tentatively—into these discussions with an almost exclusive focus on media representations of concussion and controversies surrounding the long-term effects of traumatic brain injury. Problematically, however, the voices of people who have experienced these injuries are largely absent from concussion research across academic disciplines. The first-person knowledge, stories, and ideas of injured persons are not well-represented within the vast body of research exploring post-concussion symptoms, mechanisms of injury, prevention strategies, treatment protocols, and, to a much lesser extent, power dynamics shaping concussion research and injury experiences. These types of studies cement the dominance of scholarly "expertise," especially knowledge rooted in biomedical fields (Malcolm 2017). This is not so different from approaches to pain and injury more generally, topics in both academic and popular literature that have been historically dominated by biomedical knowledges (Burkitt 1999; Bendelow and Williams 1995; Morris 1991; Williams and Bendelow 1998). Within scientific paradigms focusing on injury diagnosis and treatment, biomedical expertise tends to take precedence over athletes' first-hand knowledge of their own experiences.

Our goal in this chapter is to follow scholars who have sought to wrest the privileged form of knowledge about concussion away from biomedical fields, arguing in our case that youth athletes' experiences and ideas are an integral aspect of contemporary "concussion knowledge." To do so, we bring youth athletes' concussion experiences into conversation with the small body of previously published work that has included participants' narratives about sport-related concussion (Caron et al. 2013; Liston et al. 2016; Malcolm 2009; Safai 2003). To expand on this previous work and with a particular focus on youth athletes' constructions of the impacts of concussion on quality of life, simultaneous feelings of interpersonal support and "aloneness," and loss of identity, we borrow from Michael Bury's original concept of "biographical disruption" and scholars who have sought to expand on his work.

Emerging out of his research with people's experiences of rheumatoid arthritis, Bury (1982, 168) suggested that a biographical disruption "highlights the resources (cognitive and material) available to individuals, modes of explanation for pain and suffering, continuities and discontinuities between professional and lay thought, and sources of variation in experience," resulting in a rupture in routine and life as people know it. Put another way, the disruption brings into question taken-for-granted assumptions about one's short- and long-term health expectations, one's relationship to their body, and the use of resources available (e.g., financial, time, social networks).

While Bury's original concept has been applied in an array of research exploring people's experiences of a variety of illnesses and chronic conditions, the concept of biographical disruption has also been used to conceptualize adults' experiences of brain injury (Sveen et al. 2016) as well as sport-related injury (Malcolm and Pullen 2018). Importantly, more recent iterations of Bury's concept have highlighted the need to expand on the idea of disrupted biographies with more careful consideration of the influence of sociocultural context on individual experience (e.g., Harris 2009; Malcolm and Pullen 2018; Sveen et al. 2016; Williams 2001). Sveen and colleagues (2016), for example, contended that the so-called disruption is but the first experience, from which adults then learn to adjust, and reconstruct new ideas about themselves and their lives in relation to their illness or injury and the larger cultural context. Harris (2009), based on research of people's experiences of their hepatitis C diagnoses, similarly argued that the experience of biographical disruption is always contextual, dependent upon many factors including previous illness experiences, community membership and norms, and influence of medical expertise.

It is the more nuanced or complex understanding of biographical disruptions provided by scholars, such as Sveen and colleagues, as well as the application of the concept to sport-related injury (Malcolm and Pullen 2018) that influences our work here, in particular given our focus on young athletes as well as our interest in complicating biomedical approaches to concussion and concussion recovery. For example, whereas neuropsychologists are typically concerned with how a patient's mental and emotional well-being influences their recovery from brain injury, our analysis explores how individual experiences of injury and recovery are connected to social norms and values within sport and beyond, with a particular interest in examining how the medicalization of concussion can downplay the importance of emotional/lived experiences of this type of injury (Malcolm 2017). While critically interrogating the experience of sport-related concussion, we have sought to foreground young people's voices within the analysis, thus positioning lived experiences as essential, but largely overlooked, components of concussion knowledge. We argue that foregrounding athletes' stories can produce different—but no less valuable—knowledge about how social norms and power structures shape what concussion "feels like" in ways not immediately accessible through medicalized treatment plans and scientific protocols.

Notes on Method

Canadian youth who were taking part in a university-led randomized controlled trial (RCT) were interviewed for this paper. The RCT began in 2017 and, at time of the writing of this chapter, was ongoing. In brief, the RCT sought to investigate the potential benefits of different forms of rehabilitation strategies (low-level aerobic exercise versus cervicovestibular rehabilitation in isolation or combination) following diagnoses of a sport-related concussion. All of the participants had symptoms for greater than 10 days following their concussion. We conducted pre- and post-treatment semi-structured interviews with both female and male participants, pursuing two general objectives: (1) to gather feedback from the athletes about the intervention itself for the benefit of the researchers and practitioners involved with the RCT and (2) to understand more about the experiences of sport-related concussion from injured persons themselves. The goal of the latter was to provide an opportunity for the "folk wisdom" (Malcolm 2017) of concussion to be gained and to contrast this embodied knowledge to the dominant medico-scientific conceptions of brain injury and recovery.

All interviews lasted approximately 30 minutes, with some lasting as long as 45 minutes. Since participants in the pre-intervention stage were still experiencing similar and varying symptoms such as dizziness, nausea, sensitivity to light and/or noise, difficulty concentrating, and irritability, every effort was made to make these young athletes as comfortable as possible during the interviews. For example, some asked for the lights to be dimmed, which was accommodated. We also made it clear that they could take breaks as needed and could also end the interviews whenever they felt that they had had enough. All managed these interviews well with some commenting that they felt grateful for the opportunity to share their stories.

All interviews were audio recorded, professionally transcribed, then analyzed thematically. We first searched for themes related specifically to our research questions but then followed the tenets of open-coding (Charmaz 2006; Saldana 2003), where we allowed ourselves to remain open to the possibility of other themes emerging out of our initial analysis. This led us, for example, to create a theme we entitled "medical care," a theme distinct from participants' opinions about the clinical intervention itself. We then created sub-themes in each of the initial codes that had been created in order to better capture the nuances and complexities of the participants' narratives, noting points of similarities and difference. While not monolithic, there were many points of overlap and convergence in these young athletes' experiences and their ideas about sport-related concussion, pain, and injury, which we discuss in this chapter: types and impacts of symptoms; frustration in relation to and distinct from support; aloneness; and a sense of a loss of identity during their concussion experiences. Many of the participants also reported similar experiences in relation to the medical system and feeling "lost" within it from time of injury to enrolment in the clinical trial (Kelly et al., 2018).

The Participants

Our interviews were conducted with 16 youth, ranging in age from 12 to 16. Nine of the participants identified as female, seven as male.[1] When asked about sport participation, the majority noted that they participated in more than one sport, but the most common sports indicated were cheerleading, field hockey, football, ice hockey, motocross, rodeo/trick riding, rugby, ski racing, soccer, swimming, tennis, and ultimate Frisbee. Secondary sports included athletics (track & field), basketball, lacrosse, triathlon, and volleyball. For most, their primary sport participation took place outside of school, but many commented that their secondary (and sometimes tertiary sports) were school-related, either intramural or inter-scholastic.

More than half of the participants reported having been diagnosed with more than one concussion in their lifetime and most had received at least one diagnosed concussion in their primary sport. That many participants had experienced a concussion in their primary sport, which represent an array of sport types, challenges popular ideas of the kind of sports in which concussions are sustained; this also suggests a need to broaden research, which to this point in time has tended to focus on contact sports almost entirely. Many of the participants also spoke of other head injuries during their athletic careers but noted they had not sought out medical treatment; as such, they were reluctant to classify them as concussions even if the symptoms were consistent with what they were experiencing as part of the diagnosed concussion that brought them into the RCT. Some, but not all, were hoping to return to their primary sport after they had fully recovered. Pseudonyms have been assigned to provide these young people with as much anonymity as possible; other identifying characteristics have also been altered or removed.

Post-Concussion Experiences and Their Impacts

Almost every participant commented that they were experiencing concussion symptoms prior to their diagnoses by medical professionals, but not all had immediately ceased sport participation at the time of the injury. In some cases, they did not seek out medical treatment until several days later when symptoms had not subsided or, in some cases, had gotten worse. Many also commented that based on what they now know about concussion, they suspected that they had had at least one concussion prior to the injury for which they were currently seeking treatment. There were also, despite the different ways that they had experienced head trauma, quite similar descriptions of their symptoms: headaches, dizziness, nausea, difficulty focusing, tiredness/fatigue but at the same time difficulty sleeping, and sensitivity to light and/or sound. The following excerpts capture the various symptoms that the participants described:

> Headache, blurred vision, not dizziness but unstable. Those were the mains. And neck pain. . . . I was feeling really good the first two days but then I got really sick and had to go to the hospital.
>
> (Dave, 16)

> [I had] light sensitivity. . . . I'm constantly tired [which is] worse in the afternoon. . . . I can fall asleep quickly, well I can't fall asleep that quickly, but I go to sleep early and then wake up like five times throughout the night. . . . It's also harder to remember stuff.
>
> (Debbie, 12)

The symptoms described by the 16 participants are largely consistent with the 22 symptoms listed on the fifth edition of the Sport Concussion Assessment Tool (SCAT5) and the Concussion Recognition Tool (CRT5). Both documents, produced out of the fifth international conference on sport-related concussion held in Berlin, Germany, in October 2016, are meant to assist in the evaluation of potential concussion; the former is directed at physicians and licensed health care professionals and the latter for other individuals such as athletic trainers, coaches, and (ostensibly) parents/guardians. The symptoms described are also similar to symptoms reported by participants in other research on sport-related concussion (e.g., Caron et al. 2013; Liston et al. 2016). While the different symptoms listed on the SCAT5 are used by medical professionals to diagnose concussion, these symptoms have far wider-reaching impacts.

The young athletes we interviewed spoke with varying degrees of openness about the ways that they felt their concussion had impacted them emotionally. Many spoke about frustration, irritability, increased likelihood of crying over often trivial matters, and loss of temper. While these outbursts could be written off as "teens being teens," the emotions that participants connected to their concussions are, we feel, imperative to note in particular since many of the participants constructed their emotions and emotional experiences as something being "completely out of their control." Moreover, they were quite forthcoming with the fact that, to greater or lesser extents, these emotional experiences impacted their relationships with others. The following interview excerpts capture many of these ideas.

> I get really annoyed with [my sister] a lot of the time because she . . . either she won't do something she's supposed to do and I will get in trouble for her not doing her chores or whatever. She'll argue about it

and stuff but I get more annoyed about it, just frustrated over it and stuff like that.

(Raj, 16)

I've been more irritated and just kind of upset with a lot of things. Things that really shouldn't upset me I just kind of, little things like a friend telling you that they're busy or something. It's like, "Oh. Okay. You're busy. Whatever." But now it's like, "Oh. I'm not good enough." Stuff like that. It's just kind of amplified. . . . It's just kind of there. Like sometimes when I should be upset I'm quite happy and it's completely reversed. Then other times I'll be talking to a friend and just remember something and it's just done. I can't control it. It wasn't even that bad; it just brings me down I guess.

(Paolo, 16)

I get frustrated more often so we've definitely fought a little more. [My mother] feels bad. Yeah. . . . I can't do anything. I don't know. It definitely comes from that. . . . There was one time I was taking a nap because it's the only thing I can do. They woke me up but to tell me there was dinner. I was so mad that they woke me up that I lost it on both of them. Then I felt terrible after. I'm like, "Oh my gosh. I feel so sorry." Yeah.

(Carolina, 16)

I've never really been anxious or nervous about stuff, but I don't know, I seem to be more anx . . . not nervous. I don't really get nervous about anything but a lot of the time I get anxious about even just simple stuff, like being on time when I'll clearly be on. . . . I don't know. I got anxious about it when I'll be 20 minutes early. I'll still worry about getting there on time and stuff like that or be anxious about getting there on time.

(Raj, 16)

I just feel a bit more on edge a lot of the time. And definitely have more anxiety than I used to. Used to have low anxiety and then suddenly I'm worrying about everything so that's probably been the biggest change for my day-to-day life. I get a lot more nervous about everything even though I know my teachers are totally supportive of me having a concussion and are willing to make extensions and to help me through it.

(Karine, 15)

I find I'm more annoyed with people. I get irritated more easily. I feel that disturbs my relationships with people, but I just let them know I'm sorry I'm this way. I've been recovering from the concussion . . . and . . . yeah.

(Kate, 16)

While in this chapter we have not focused on parent/guardian interviews that were also conducted as part of this project, here we want to highlight the consensus amongst the adults that concussion had coincided with altered and sometimes (as they constructed it) "irrational behaviour" of their children. One parent spoke about her son's increased emotional state, for example, noting that he cried more since his concussion. The son of which this parent spoke also commented on the fact that he had been crying more than usual but then also noted there were issues with a romantic partner that were causing that. He did not (or had not) made the connection between his concussion, the symptoms he was experiencing, and relationship difficulties, but it is difficult not to infer at least some correlation, especially since most of the participants spoke about the various relationship difficulties they had been experiencing while dealing with the more "physical" post-concussion symptoms. The difficulties these young athletes were experiencing with others in their lives mirror personal relationship challenges discussed by (retired) athletes and their partners, a topic of both academic and media discourse (see, e.g., Caron et al. 2013; Ciskie 2012; Kelly 2018; TSN Staff 2018). The significant difference, of course, is the age of our participants and their limited life experiences.

Some athletes specifically connected their feelings—sadness and anger especially—to the fact that they were not able to participate in sport. Rather than perceiving it as a symptom of the concussion, it was constructed more as what the concussion had resulted in: exclusion from a space that provided them social networks, physical activity, the opportunity to excel, and a sense of self-identity intricately connected to sport participation and (more often than not) winning. The following three interview excerpts demonstrate the prevalence of this sort of narrative across ages, gender, and type of sport.

> I felt really hurt inside, just because I can't do it. It almost made me feel "less," I guess. And sad because I won't be able to do it for a little bit, just so I do heal up properly this time.
>
> (Beth, 14)

> I was pretty sad but that was probably because I'm a people person and I was stuck in a room by myself for four days. [Sport] is part of who I am, almost. I play a lot of sports.
>
> (Kara, 16)

> I get angry more often now. That's it though. I just get angry. With everyone. I just love sports. It's like everything in my life is sports. It's just . . . Yeah. So, when I can't do sports it's pretty terrible.
>
> (Mark, 13)

In most instances, we were interviewing these youth athletes while they were still experiencing many of their post-concussion symptoms and, as such, they were able to explain what they were physically feeling and also articulate the ways these symptoms were impacting their lives in—perhaps to them— unexpected ways. That similar symptoms and their impacts have been reported in qualitative research on sport- and non-sport related concussion (Caron et al. 2013; Cassilo and Sanderson 2018; Iadevaia et al. 2015; Liston et al. 2016) speaks to some universality in concussion experiences, even if gender, age, mechanism of injury, individual symptoms, diagnosis, and treatment protocol may vary. This adds some complexity to the notion that every concussion is unique, an idea frequently put forth by medical practitioners and clinicians. If the neurobiological and neuro-psychological trajectories are always unique to each individual, the fact that there is so much commonality in terms of social/emotional experiences speaks to the influence of the larger cultural context and—in this case—sport, more specifically, on individual experiences.

Frustration and (Lack of) Support

> It's frustrating, not riding. That's definitely it. Not being able to ride. That's a big way to get rid of stress and all that, and when I can't ride, I get cranky. . . . This is the prime riding time right now, so just not being able to ride, that really has affected my mood and all that.
>
> (Peter, 13)

Similar to individuals interviewed by other scholars in their research on sport- and non-sport related concussion (Caron et al. 2013; Iadevaia et al. 2015; Liston et al. 2016), there was an overwhelming sense of frustration evident in the athletes' stories shared with us. These frustrations resulted, as in the quote from Peter above, from their inability to participate in sport, their struggle with academic tasks, challenges within familial relationships, and isolation from their social networks, in sport and at school. There was certainly also a sense of frustration that emerged in connection to what was constructed as a shift in emotionality and a perceived lack of control in relation to emotions. Frustration was also evident in the length of time athletes felt that it would take them to return to sport, if they were to return at all—an important point, to which we will return later in the chapter.

When the topic of support was raised, it was largely framed in a positive way when the athletes perceived that friends, family, coaches, and/or teachers understood what the athletes were going through. Support was constructed as being evident when athletes were made to still feel part of their team or training environment, when they felt that coaches had their best interests at heart (i.e., not pushing them back to the field of play), when family members asked how they were doing and did not pressure them to do things that they were not comfortable with, and when teachers made special arrangements for school work—including homework, assignments, and tests. The following interview excerpts are representative of these different ideas about support and support that was constructed as positive.

[My friends] are really scared for me because they want me back for the summer, but I don't know. They're making sure I don't do anything stupid.

(Beth, 16)

It hasn't really affected it [relationship with teammates] that much. They've just been sympathetic. The quarterback was upset that I was missing games but he's not really, I'm not really friends with him. . . . People are concerned about it. My teammates and friends were surprised how long it's lasting. . . . They're understanding and okay with it. I even tried to come back one day and they wouldn't let me without a doctor's consent.

(Raj, 16)

My coach just wants to follow-up with me because I was doing so . . . I think he's fine with it pretty much. We've had concussions in our group before.

(Celine, 13)

My relationship with my parents is pretty good. I'm really close with my dad because we have a lot of things in common and he's more interested in the things I'm interested. [My mom] is really supportive. She's pretty anxious about things or she wants everything to be neat and tidy all the time but that's how it's always been from the start. But I think they both understand that I feel a little bit not myself because of my concussion. So, my relationship with them hasn't really changed too much.

(Karine, 15)

My mom is really helpful. If I'm just completely, like I can't do anything at that point, she's just like, "Alright, I'll come and pick you up" or something like that and I just go home or something like that.

(Paolo, 16)

My teachers have been super supportive, especially my math teacher because I think she's had a background with concussions and she was talking to me and said, "You know what, just take it as slow as you need to; we'll talk about when we need to get back or what you need to catch up on, but right now don't do anything that you're not comfortable with." So, she was really good. And all my other teachers, because I get along slower . . . so in drama I had to give a speech and I could not remember anything I was supposed to say and the teacher just told me "don't do that." And even on other things, when I had to write essays for

English, I got extensions because I just had trouble typing or looking at computer screens for a long time.

(Karine, 15)

Some of the athletes' narratives, however, were not so "neat and tidy," as reflected in Dave's comment related to school:

Teachers get that I have a concussion, but they don't get that I can't do anything with . . . they treat me well in class, they don't make me do things in class, but then they expect me to get the work done somehow. And that's the part that I don't get. They're good to me in class, like, "Oh, you don't have to do this, you don't have to do that. Don't take those notes." But then when they hand out a worksheet, they're like, "Just complete it whenever" and I feel like that's unrealistic to keep giving me worksheets that I can't complete right now. Expecting to complete them later.

(Dave, 16)

While beyond the scope of our work here, Dave's point does raise an important issue of how teachers are left with little understanding of how to work with students post-concussion, a line of research and praxis that desperately needs to be undertaken.

Two of our participants also described how parents refused to believe that their child was injured, insisting that the post-concussion symptoms were not "real" or that their child was "faking it."

[My dad] doesn't believe I have a concussion. I don't know, he's weird about that stuff. He's always been like that. He [was sick] and he went to work all the time, so . . . I don't feel pressured by him to like get better faster but I feel like he doesn't really believe me. I don't know, it's hard to say. He's like, "I went to work when I [was sick]". It's not pressure to get better faster, it's just a little bit of guilt.

(Dave, 16)

My dad's just like, "Oh well." He thinks I'm faking, so I don't know. He's like, "What are you complaining for?" I'm like, "Yeah, 'cause I was tired." He's like, "It makes it seem like you want to quit." I'm like, "I don't want to quit. What?!" My dad's interesting with this. When I said this week again that I didn't want to go to practice, he wanted me to go back to practice and I had a headache so I didn't go. My dad was like, "Oh well . . . makes it seem like you want to quit. It doesn't seem like you're really focused on [your sport] anymore." Then I'm like, "I am. I'm just sore and they told me not to come back if I have headaches."

(Celine, 13)

That both Dave and Celine made it quite clear in these interview excerpts that they were speaking specifically about their fathers can be interpreted in relation to dominant gender norms, particularly in what has been a well-researched connection between traditional masculine norms and health. Scholars have argued that socially constructed norms lead men to be less likely to speak openly about health issues (see, e.g., Addis and Mahalik 2003; Courtenay 2000; Dumas and Bournival 2012; Gough 2006) and to adopt a "push through pain" mentality reflective of hyper-masculinity and machismo argued to be common in the context of most sporting spaces (see, e.g., Caron et al. 2013; Messner 1990; Young et al. 1995). The articulation of these masculine norms through the comments from Dave and Celine can be directly contrasted to their perceptions of their mothers as supportive, if not overly-cautious, about their return to sport. In general, there were several instances in which our participants described how positive experiences of support were also entangled with (internal and external) pressure to "get back to normal." These conflicting messages demonstrate how experiences of concussion can be characterized by multiple and often competing sets of emotions that may shape an athlete's relationship with their sports, loved ones, and their world-view more broadly.

Isolation, Aloneness, and Loss of Identity

Many of the young athletes spoke quite openly about a sense of isolation or "aloneness" that characterized their concussion experiences. This sense of aloneness emerged in reference to literal isolation in dark rooms immediately following their experience of head trauma, a commonly prescribed treatment through their initial encounters with medical professionals and/or self-prescribed based on their knowledge at the time. This sense of aloneness also often related to a (perceived) lack of support from other individuals in these young athletes' lives, as described in the preceding section.

There was also a sense of frustration and aloneness communicated by participants in relation to the idea that concussion is considered and popularly referred to as an "invisible" injury. While people can (seek to) describe their symptoms, concussion nevertheless remains something that is unseen by others: there are no crutches, no braces, no wrappings, no kinesthetic tape. And yet there remains an experience of the world as an "injured person," complicated by the important role that sport can play in people's lives and in constructing their sense of identity. In this vein, many of the athletes we interviewed also described how through the initial injury and the lingering impacts, they lost their sense of who they were and their sense of their place in the world.

> The one thing that bothers me a lot is because I'm used to winning stuff, I guess, and I know I'm not going to be doing that.
>
> (Celine, 13)

Hockey's my life. It's pretty bad. I live for hockey. It's just my favourite thing to do, still. I just love everything about it. In our school, it's like status. Hockey players are at the top. It just means like you're the cool kids, you're the popular kids, kind of. [I fear] that I might have to stop playing sports.

(Mark, 13)

I'm playing a pretty high level, right, and then I couldn't play. I could play if I wanted to, next year, and then go play on one [team] where everybody's really big, everybody's really fast, in the hockey that I want to play. But obviously, there's hitting. I can go play rec, which is still fun hockey, but right now, I really like the challenge of hockey. While I think it would be really fun to go play rec, I just want to feel the challenge of normal hockey. I would say I'm definitely concerned about my status. Like all my friends play high-level league. That's what we talk about, so I feel like if I played low-level, like I talk about how I score a goal against the top team now, they're like "That's sick" but then I talk about scoring a goal and then they're like "Well, everybody sucks." Who cares right? But it's obviously a status thing.

(Dave, 16)

While much could be said about the cultural capital connected to ice hockey in the Canadian context (and men's ice hockey in particular) in relation to Mark and Dave's comments above, we are more interested in the general sense of "loss of identity" that was prevalent in many of the athletes' narratives. Many of these young athletes commented in various ways on a loss of identity in the short term. But, given the uncertainty around the length and success of their recovery, participants also communicated concerns about their future as an athlete. Many of our participants' comments show them to be grappling with the possibility that they would not be able to participate in the same way—if at all—in a sport that they love and consider a central part of who they are. These feelings were likely reinforced through (perceived) pressure from teammates, coaches, and parents to return to sport, especially if the athletes' potential return to play was believed to be directly connected to the success of the team.

Everybody was, like, sad. Because it was playoffs time. And we were on a roll then . . . we were gonna' win the playoffs. I played every game up until we made it to semifinal and we lost the semifinal and I wasn't there. And then we were on the winning side, so with that we dropped down to the loser's bracket semifinal and we lost that one too. So, everybody was sad. I was leading on the team, so there's like a couple of situations. We went to a shootout in one game and I always go in the shootout, but I wasn't there. So, people were just sad that I didn't get the chance to win and see the championships. But yeah. They were sad for me but they also want me to be better. Yeah, they want to win more than they want me not to have a concussion. They kinda' wanted me to play.

(Dave, 16)

My team isn't happy. Not great. I was one of the better players on it I think. According to the coaches. My coaches ask me about starting to play again, but they're supposed to. But in a practice, I was asked to head the ball about a week after I first visited the concussion place.

(Debbie, 13)

What is troubling about these quotes and the larger narrative from which they are drawn, is that these young athletes' ideas don't sound much different from how older and/or professional athletes have spoken about the pressure that they felt to "return to play" following a concussion. For example, in interviews with retired NHL players who had experienced multiple concussions, Caron and colleagues (2013) note that the league promoted a sense of "playing through pain" that impacted players' treatment protocols and decision to return to the game—in many cases—prematurely. This is not so different from empirical research on sport-related pain and injury more generally: a significant body of literature produced over the past 40 years has suggested that elite sport promotes a "no pain, no gain" philosophy, which can create and work to maintain a culture of silence in relation to pain and injury. Moreover, across different sports and at different levels, scholars have noted athletes' relationships to pain as an effect of over-conformity to, or normalization of, athletic discourses (Atkinson 2008; Bridel 2013; Hughes and Coakley 1991; Noe 1973; Theberge 2008). Perhaps not surprisingly then, some of the athletes also seemed to place pressure on themselves to return as quickly as possible to the field of play not just because they missed participating in their chosen sport(s) but because they perceived themselves to be a key player on their team. As one 13-year-old basketball player commented in no uncertain terms, "I am the best."

Contrary to previous sport-related pain and injury research, some of our participants also commented that head injuries weren't being ignored or normalized. To borrow from Safai's (2003) work, there was evidence of a "culture of precaution" in these athletes' experiences, including from coaches, parents, teammates, teachers, and the athletes themselves. We suggest that this likely reflects a general increased awareness about concussion through various educational campaigns within sport and the media, education which carries, amongst other themes, a message of "urgency" when head trauma is involved; coverage of high-profile athletes and TBI certainly contributes to this construction of concussion as a continued considerable concern (Malcolm 2017) with more conservative attitudes emerging even in the most surprising of places: the NFL (Anderson and Kian 2012). Malcolm (2009) has also suggested, however, that cautionary approaches can be related to uncertainty on the part of sport medicine practitioners in terms of diagnosis and/or treatment of concussion since much remains unknown, even across contemporary research findings. As he asserts, there is much debate among scientists about how to define "concussion" and standardize treatment protocols; yet Malcolm also describes a general sense of confusion contributing to practitioners' fear of having their knowledge about diagnosis and treatment undermined by others.

Conceptualizing Concussion as an "Athletic Disruption"

There is, of course, a great deal of complexity in our participants' experiences of concussion and the way they talked about these experiences. Their accounts were by no means monolithic and cannot be reduced to a singular point of analysis. To do so would negate the messiness of their singular and collective experiences. While no "one" concussion story emerged from our interviews, however, the similarity and overlap in experiences of frustration, aloneness, and loss of identity following injury diagnosis and—to different extents—throughout the recovery process, were striking.

Scholars have argued that in most scenarios pain complicates the ways that people think about their bodies and complicates their ideas about their identity (Leder 1990; Morris 1991; Scarry 1985; Williams and Bendelow 1998). This has the result of disrupting people's "biographies, selves, and the taken-for-granted structures of the world upon which they rest" (Williams and Bendelow 1998, 159). In sport, however, it has been argued that experiences of pain seem to draw people closer to their bodies and closer to their selves. Recognizing the pervasiveness of pain, in fact, is important since it seems that the ability to endure it, tolerate it, overcome it becomes a significant way that sport participants come to identify themselves (Bale 2004, 2006; Loland 2006; Young 2004) and an athletic performance for which they are rewarded by others. While experiences of pain can work to alienate people from their bodies, they can at the same time work to remind individuals of their corporeality (Bruhm 1994; Leder 1990; Scarry 1985). Put another way, experiences of pain are one way that people come to constitute themselves as embodied subjects while simultaneously calling into question how people think about themselves, their bodies, and their place in the world. Our participants' responses express how concussion may engender similar contradictions.

That young athletes conceptualized their experience of concussion as disruptive to their sense of self is consistent with the popular idea that athletic involvement and achievement can be a key part of identity formation. In ways similar to persons with chronic illness who feel uncertain about their futures (e.g., Bury 1982; Harris 2009), the young athletes in our study often spoke specifically about or alluded to the idea of uncertainty. Beyond simply being immobilized to varying degrees because of the physical symptoms they were experiencing, many participants communicated feeling emotionally arrested by questions of "why?", "what if?", "what next?", and "who am I without sport?" These youth seemed to be stuck in liminal space, a space betwixt and between, a space of great uncertainty.

This is not so different from what Malcolm and Pullen (2018) argued, using Bury's concept; they asserted that sport-related injuries can be understood as a particular type of biographical disruption that while not particularly serious in terms of one's immediate health circumstances, nevertheless forces the cessation of people's "normalized" activities and embodied practices, calling future health status into question. They wrote, "The resultant estrangement [participants] experienced from these highly meaningful social experiences was particularly difficult to overcome because in many cases exercise was a strategy deliberately evoked to manage future health uncertainties" (p. 15). For our young athletes, however, it was likely less a consideration of future health "uncertainties" and more about the immediate and (potential) future impact on sport participation—something which was constructed as being of great importance to their present and future sense of self-identity.

These fears, we suggest, speak to the power of sport discourse, which seems to permeate all levels of play. The intensity of athletes' self-identification with dominant sporting values has been highlighted in previous research as an explanation for why athletes might try to hide or downplay potential concussion symptoms (and other injuries more generally): playing with pain and injury is socially valued because it shows commitment to the game (Liston et al. 2016) and, we would add, one's worthiness of the "athlete" label. If one connects their sense of self to this label—seemingly irrespective of age and/or level of sport—and are told that they cannot play for an undetermined amount of time, then their lived experience forcefully disrupts the story they have told, and tell about, themselves. Thus, following from calls to further contextualize the notion of biographical disruption while also accounting for the meaning and originary status of experience (Scott 1991), these young athletes' constructions of concussion and a total loss of identity suggests more an "athletic disruption"—or a disruption in the creation and maintenance of their "athletic identity." While it is perhaps difficult for youth (and adults, for that matter) to disentangle a disruption to their athletic self from their holistic self (i.e., distinguishing between an athletic and a biographical disruption) this is an important consideration for people in the lives of these individuals—that is, to recognize what (in our case) youth athletes' may be struggling with beyond the "physical" symptoms of concussion.

To be clear, in offering athletic disruption as a subset of biographical disruption if you will, we are not seeking to critique youths' ideas that they shared with us but rather provide statement on the continued need to critique and challenge the pervasiveness of dominant sport discourse through which our participants—and athletes more generally—make sense of themselves and the world around them. Organized sport is a social space that predominantly promotes winning over wellness, a notion built around the masculine glorification of toughness and pain, as well as medical practices that may prioritize fitness to compete over short- or long-term health (Safai 2003; Theberge 2008; Waddington 2004). Yet the contemporary public concern about concussion has interrupted many prevailing cultural scripts around what it means to an athlete, especially the construction of injuries as adversity best overcome through hard work, determination, and the vanquishing of pain. As media representations have become spaces for dissemination of athletes' stories of concussion and the potentially lingering, disruptive consequences of these injuries (Ventresca 2019), many of these portrayals run counter to widespread celebratory narratives created around athletes' abilities to overcome and/or play through injury (Anderson and Kian 2012). Thus, the intensity of the athletic disruptions associated with concussion may stem from the ineffectiveness of traditional sports values to help athletes make sense of their injury and recovery as well as their (sometimes questionable) return to sport.

Concluding Thoughts

In this chapter, we have used qualitative materials gathered through semi-structured interviews with young athletes to think critically about sport-related concussion. Through thematic analysis of the materials, we were able to gain a sense of the kinds of physical symptoms our participants were experiencing (or had experienced), as well as the impact of these symptoms on emotional and relational experiences. Throughout we have argued the necessity of including injured persons' lived experiences as an integral part of concussion knowledge moving forward.

Foregrounding participants' experiences may be novel in much of the body of research on sport-related concussion, but it is by no means uncharted territory. Such an approach follows from the legacy of the women's health movement and scholarship within critical disability studies. Both examples are powerful reminders of the ways "voices" and experiences can and should be central to the production of knowledge. In the 1990s, for example, disability scholars and activists rallied around the notion of "nothing about us, without us," chipping away at the medical model of disability, a model that reproduced an expert/dependent binary and paternalistic attitudes toward persons with impairments (e.g., Charlton 1998; Shakespeare 2014, 2017). These historical examples demonstrate how patients' voices can make important contributions to the diagnoses and treatment process as well as policy development and implementation, thereby wresting sole authority (i.e., power) away from the biomedical field. In sum, we assert through our work here that there is great potential in making the lived experiences of those with concussion and post-concussion symptoms central to the production of "concussion knowledge."

We have also argued for the need to contextualize concussion experiences, using our interpretation of Bury's concept of biographical disruption as a way to conceptualize peoples' experiences of sport-related concussion. In the contemporary sociocultural context, biomedical knowledge about concussion too often is positioned as the "Truth" despite continued uncertainty about what constitutes effective diagnosis and treatment, as well as how to define the long-term consequences of these injuries (Malcolm 2017; Ventresca 2019). Moreover, sport-related concussion is often presented as being of paramount concern within sport but also as something that can be "fixed" by/through biomedical and technological interventions exclusively, an idea which seems to preclude the need to think critically about the culture of sport while upholding so-called positive physical, mental, and social benefits of sport participation. The notion of "athletic disruption" reflects the disruptive potential of brain injuries whilst also highlighting the pervasiveness of sport discourse in these young athlete's understanding of themselves and their place in the world. Such knowledge helps us to complicate an exclusive "diagnosis and treatment" approach to sport-related concussion, as is the case with a purely biomedical focus on concussion. Such approaches fail to address concussion holistically, including the athletic disruption in these young people's lives, the articulation of this disruption with their overall sense of self, and the potential impact such disruptive experiences may have on individual recovery.

Note

1. Information gathered on the youth participants focused on sex, age, and physical characteristics such as weight and height. This information was deemed as what was necessary for intake into the RCT. Given the type and number of sports that the youth participated in as well as that they were able to access clinical care on a university campus suggests that they would most likely be middle class, but—importantly—that involves speculation on our part and should be considered a limitation of our work here.

References

Addis, Michael, and James Mahalik. 2003. "Men, Masculinity, and the Contexts of Help Seeking." *American Psychologist* 58 (1): 5–14. doi:10.1037/0003-066X.58.1.5.

Anderson, Eric, and Edward Kian. 2012. "Examining Media Contestation of Masculinity and Head Trauma in the National Football League." *Men & Masculinities* 15 (2): 152–173. doi:10.1177/1097184X11430127.

Atkinson, Michael. 2008. "Triathlon, Suffering, and Exciting Significance." *Leisure Studies* 27 (2): 165–180. doi:10.1080/02614360801902216.

Bale, John. 2004. *Running Cultures: Racing in Time and Space.* London: Routledge.

Bale, John. 2006. "The Place of Pain in Running." In *Pain and Injury in Sport: Social and Ethical Analysis,* edited by Sigmund Loland, Berit Skirstad & Ivan Waddington. 65–75. New York: Routledge.

Bendelow, Gillian, and Simon Williams. 1995. "Transcending the Dualisms: Towards a Sociology of Pain." *Sociology of Health and Illness* 17 (2): 139–165. https://doi.org/10.1111/j.1467-9566.1995.tb00479.x

Benson, Peter. 2017. "Big Football: Corporate Social Responsibility and the Culture and Color of Injury in America's Most Popular Sport." *Journal of Sport and Social Issues* 41 (4): 307–334. doi:10.1177/0193723517707699.

Bridel, William. 2013. "Not Fat, Not Skinny, Functional Enough to Finish: Interrogating Constructions of Health in the Ironman Triathlon." *Leisure/Loisir* 37 (1): 37–56. doi:10.1080/14927713.2013.776745.

Bruhm, Steven. 1994. *Gothic Bodies: The Politics of Pain in Romantic Fiction.* Philadelphia: University of Pennsylvania Press.

Burkitt, Ian. 1999. *Bodies of Thought: Embodiment, Identity and Modernity.* London: Sage.

Bury, Michael. 1982. "Chronic Illness as Biographical Disruption." *Sociology of Health and Illness* 4 (2): 167–182. doi:10.1111/1467-9566.ep11339939.

Caron, Jeff, Gordon Bloom, Karen Johnston, and Catherine Sabiston. 2013. "Effects of Multiple Concussions on Retired National Hockey League Players." *Journal of Sport & Exercise Psychology* 35: 168–179. doi:10.1123/jsep.35.2.168.

Cassilo, David, and Jimmy Sanderson. 2018. "From Social Isolation to Becoming an Advocate: Exploring Athletes' Grief Discourse About Lived Concussion Experiences in Online Forums." *Communication & Sport.* Advance online publication. doi:10.1177/2167479518790039.

Charlton, James. 1998. *Nothing About Us without Us: Disability Oppression and Empowerment.* Berkeley, CA: University of California Press.

Charmaz, Kathy. 2006. *Constructing Grounded Theory: A Practical Guide Through Qualitative Analysis.* Thousand Oaks: Sage.

Ciskie, Bruce. 2012. Chris Pronger's Scary Concussion, as Experienced by Wife Lauren. *SB Nation*, January 20. www.sbnation.com/nhl/2012/1/20/2719942/chris-pronger-injury-concussion-interview-philadelphia-flyers

Courtenay, Will. 2000. "Constructions of Masculinity and Their Influence on Men's Well-Being: A Theory of Gender and Health." *Social Science & Medicine* 50 (10): 1385–1401.

Dumas, Alexandre, and Bournival, Emily. 2012. "Men, Masculinities, and Health: Theory and Application." In *Men and Masculinities: An Interdisciplinary Reader*, edited by Jason Laker, 32–47. Don Mills, ON: Oxford University Press.

Gough, Brendan. 2006. "Try to Be Healthy, But Don't Forgo Your Masculinity: Deconstructing Men's Health Discourse in the Media." *Social Science & Medicine* 63 (9): 2476–2488. doi:10.1016/j.socscimed.2006.06.004.

Harris, Magdalena. 2009. "Troubling Biographical Disruption: Narratives of Unconcern about Hepatitis C Diagnosis." *Sociology of Health & Illness* 31 (7): 1028–1042. doi:10.1111/j.1467–9566.2009.01172.x.

Hughes, Robert, and Jay Coakley. 1991. "Positive Deviance Among Athletes: The Implications of Overconformity to the Sport Ethic." *Sociology of Sport Journal* 8, 307–325. doi:10.1123/ssj.8.4.307.

Iadevaia, Cheree, Trevor Roiger, and Mary Beth Zwart. 2015. "Qualitative Examination of Adolescent Health-Related Quality of Life at One Year Post-Concussion." *Journal of Athletic Training* 50 (11): 1182–1189. doi:10.4085/1062-6050-50.11.02.

Kelly, Danika, William Bridel, Matt Ventresca, and Kathryn Schneider. 2018. "'I Don't Actually Know When I Knew It Was a Concussion': Athletes' Experiences of Concussion and Accessing Care." *Canadian Academy of Sport and Exercise Medicine Conference (poster presentation)*. Halifax: Canada.

Kelly, Emily. 2018. "I'm the Wife of a Former NFL Player. Football Destroyed His Kind." *The New York Times*, February 2. www.nytimes.com/2018/02/02/opinion/sunday/nfl-cte-brain-damage.html.

Leder, David. 1990. *The Absent Body.* Chicago: The University of Chicago Press.

Liston, Katie, Mark McDowell, Dominic Malcolm, Andrea Scott-Bell, and Ivan Waddington. 2016. "On Being 'Head Strong': The Pain Zone and Concussion in Non-Elite Rugby Union." *International Review for the Sociology of Sport* 53 (6): 1–17. doi:10.1177/1012690216679966.

Loland, Sigmund. 2006. "Three Approaches to the Study of Pain in Sport. In *Pain and Injury in Sport: Social and Ethical Analysis*, edited by Sigmund Loland, Berit Skirstad, and Ivan Waddington, 49–62. New York: Routledge.

Malcolm, Dominic. 2009. "Medical Uncertainty and Clinician-Athlete Relations: The Management of Concussion Injuries in Rugby Union." *Sociology of Sport Journal* 26 (2): 191–210. doi:10.1123/ssj.26.2.191.

Malcolm, Dominic. 2017. *Sport, Medicine, and Health: The Medicalization of Sport?* London: Routledge.

Malcolm, Dominic, and Emma Pullen. 2018. "Everything I Enjoy Doing I Just Couldn't Do: Biographical Disruptions for Sport-Related Injury." *Health*, 1–18. doi:10.1177/1363459318800142.

Maloney, Tom. 2016. "Hockey, Concussions, and the Media." In *How Canadians Communicate V: Sports*, edited by David Taras, and Christopher Waddell, 195–208. Edmonton: Athabasca University Press.

Messner, Michael. 1990. "When Bodies are Weapons: Masculinity and Violence in Sport." *International Review for the Sociology of Sport* 25 (3): 203–219. doi:10.1177/101269029002500303.

Morris, David. 1991. *The Culture of Pain*. Berkeley: University of California Press.

Noe, Francis. 1973. "Coaches, Players, and Pain." *International Review for the Sociology of Sport* 8 (2): 47–60. doi.org/10.1177/101269027300800204.

Safai, Parissa. 2003. "Healing the Body in the 'Culture of Risk': Examining the Negotiation of Treatment Between Sport Medicine Clinicians and Injured Athletes in Canadian Intercollegiate Sport. *Sociology of Sport Journal* 20 (2): 127–146. doi:10.1123/ssj.20.2.127.

Saldana, Johnny. 2003. *Longitudinal Qualitative Research: Analyzing Change Through Time*. Walnut Creek, CA: AltaMira Press.

Scarry, Elaine. 1985. *The Body in Pain: The Making and Unmaking of the World*. Oxford: Oxford University Press.

Scott, Joan. 1991. "The Evidence of Experience." *Critical Inquiry* 17 (4): 773–797.

Shakespeare, Tom. 2014. *Disability Rights and Wrongs Revisited* (2nd Ed.). London: Routledge.

Shakespeare, Tom. 2017. *Disability: The Basics*. London: Routledge.

Sveen, Unni, Helene Lundgaard Soberg, and Sigrid Ostensjo. 2016. "Biographical Disruption, Adjustment, and Reconstruction of Everyday Occupations and Work Participation after Mild Traumatic Brain Injury." *Disability & Rehabilitation* 38 (23): 2296–2304. doi:10.3109/09638288.2015.1129445.

Theberge, Nancy. 2008. "Just a Normal Bad Part of What I Do": Elite Athletes' Accounts of the Relationship Between Health and Sport. *Sociology of Sport Journal* 25 (2): 206–222. doi:10.1123/ssj.25.2.206.

TSN Staff. 2018. Franzen's Wife Details NHLer's Brain Injury. *TSN*, May 28. www.tsn.ca/wings-franzen-struggling-with-brain-injury-1.1096728.

Ventresca, Matt. 2019. "The Curious Case of CTE: Mediating Materialities of Traumatic Brain Injury." *Communication and Sport* 7 (2): 135–156. doi:10.1177/21674795186761636.

Waddington, Ivan. 2004. "Sport, Health, and Public Policy." In *Sporting Bodies, Damaged Selves: Sociological Studies in Sports-Related Injury*, edited by Kevin Young, 287–307. London: Elsevier.

Williams, Simon. 2001. "Chronic Illness as Biographical Disruption or Biographical Disruption as Chronic Illness? Reflections on a Core Concept." *Sociology of Health and Illness* 22 (1): 40–67. https://doi.org/10.1111/1467-9566.00191.

Williams, Simon, and Gillian Bendelow. 1998. *The Lived Body: Sociological Themes, Embodied Issues*. London: Routledge.

Young, Kevin. 2004. "Sports-Related Pain and Injury: Sociological Notes." In *Sporting Bodies, Damaged Selves: Sociological Studies in Sports-Related Injury*, edited by Kevin Young, 1–25. Oxford: Elsevier.

Young, Kevin, Philip White, and William McTeer. 1995. "Body Talk: Male Athletes Reflect on Sport, Injury and Pain." *Sociology of Sport Journal* 11 (2): 175–194.

7 Trauma and Recovery

Boxing and Violence Against Women in a 'Neurological Age'

Cathy van Ingen

Introduction

For the past 12 years I have been doing research and direct service work with over 1800 women who have experienced sexual assault and violence. The testimony of these participants is at the heart of much of my work, which seeks to provide a safe, trauma-informed, non-contact boxing program for women in the aftermath of violence and trauma. Those familiar with boxing know the sport's reputation as a bodily craft that places a high premium on physical force and the ability to endure physical suffering, including repetitive head trauma (Wacquant 1995). In Shape Your Life (SYL), a trauma-informed approach reconfigures the sport to a non-contact form so that it plays an important role in the lives of women *recovering* from gender-based violence. This chapter places women's experiences with trauma, violence, and boxing at the centre of analysis. It challenges assumptions about boxing as simply about violent combat that inevitably leads to brain injury. This chapter engages the scholarship and activism of feminist ideas which are central to the philosophy of SYL—and in doing so, works to disrupt some of the focus of the "neuro revolution," the increasing focus on brain science that too often obstructs the structural nature of gender-based violence and its impact on the everyday lives of women.

Boxing was the first sport where the cumulative long-term neurological effects of head trauma were recognized (Bernick and Banks 2013). What is now known as chronic traumatic encephalopathy (CTE) was first reported in medical literature in 1928 in an article titled "Punch Drunk." Pathologist Dr. Harrison Martland (1928), wrote:

> For some time fight fans and promoters have recognized a peculiar condition occurring among prize fighters which, in ring parlance, they speak of as "punch drunk." Fighters in whom the early symptoms are well recognized are said by the fans to be "cuckoo," "goofy," "cutting paper dolls," or "slug nutty."

Boxing and other combat sports continue to be important sites for studying the effects of head trauma resulting from repetitive concussive and sub-concussive blows. While the long-term neurological consequences of boxing continue to be debated, there is broad international medical consensus calling for the sport to develop increased safety measures or be abolished outright (Lundberg 1986).

Indeed, boxing has a long and complicated history as a "violent" sport. The World Medical Assembly (2017) has, for decades, called for a ban, citing that the sport's "basic intent is to produce bodily harm by specifically targeting the head." It is undeniable that boxing is a dangerous sport. However, boxing, precisely because of its intensely visceral "body-centered universe" (Wacquant 1995), can also be key to recovery from trauma. Before turning to examine the ways the SYL project uses non-contact boxing to address the trauma that is held in participant's bodies, I outline how SYL is informed by feminist trauma work. This scholarship is additionally important for critiquing the dominant medical approach to head injuries that privileges brain science over the inequities that in turn help to enable women's ongoing exposure to sexual abuse, violence, and trauma. I then more specifically discuss SYL and provide voices of the program's participants—voices that make clear trauma is not simply about injuries to brains, but is locatable in the body—and thus responses to trauma must focus on assisting survivors to reconnect with their bodies.

Feminist Trauma Work

In her groundbreaking and still relevant work, *Trauma and Recovery: The aftermath of violence—from domestic abuse to political terror*, Judith Herman argues that to study trauma and to work with survivors requires "bearing witness to horrible events" (1997, 1). This is an important premise at the root of feminist trauma work. Increasingly, however, trauma research is focused on neurobiological underpinnings and mapping the ways in which traumatic experiences produce abnormalities in the amygdala, the hippocampus, and the medial frontal cortex. Feminists working with trauma survivors are concerned with the reductionism inherent in this neurobiological explanatory trend. Specifically, a focus on the biological markers of trauma has generated concern that issues that feminists originally made visible in trauma theory, in particular the social and political contexts in which gendered violence occurs, are downplayed or ignored as neuroscientific definitions of trauma take centre stage (Tseris 2013).

Bessel Van Der Kolk (2014), a pioneering trauma researcher, asserts that we are on the verge of becoming a trauma-conscious society. Yet this notion of trauma is narrowly conceived as part of a biological process. He attributes this awareness to recent scientific advances, largely in neuroscience, that show how trauma rewires the brain. While this paradigmatic shift in trauma theory has generated new understandings and treatment methods rooted in the neurobiological basis of trauma, there is a rather paradoxical underside. Feminist scholars and activists working in trauma have long argued for a far more nuanced recognition of trauma, one that takes into account the socio-political context of women's lives, especially given the high levels of gendered violence experienced by girls and women. In *Trauma and Recovery*, Herman provides concepts for understanding, defining and treating trauma through a comprehensive approach that addresses the biological, psychological, social, and political dimensions of trauma. She rightly notes that the study of trauma "is an inherently political enterprise because it calls attention to the experience of oppressed people" (p. 237). In short, Herman's work insists that trauma has historical, social and political contexts that matter. Her book opens with a chapter titled "A Forgotten History," that traces the study of psychological trauma from early neurologists treating women's "hysteria" to "shell-shocked" veterans of both world wars, to survivors of domestic violence. Herman's scholarship on violence against women is steadfast in its focus—the study of trauma must be anchored in a context that challenges the abuses and subordination of women and children as well as the silencing and denial that surround it.

Herman extends this argument by stating that the study of trauma depends on external factors including the support of a political movement, one that radically attends to issues of power, injustice and inequality. In 2018, an evolving and increasing visible #MeToo movement signalled yet another call towards addressing sexual assault and violence directed at girls and women as well as the widespread culture that overlooks, condones and enables gender-based violence. This important issue must be addressed on multiple levels and the colossal scale of the problem of violence against girls and women has yet to be fully addressed within and through the sporting world. An article in *The Guardian* covering the sexual abuse trial of the sports doctor for the U.S. Olympic team, the United States Gymnastics Association, and Michigan State University called it the "biggest sexual abuse scandal in sports history, one whose effects will resonate for years to come" (Graham 2018). In a courtroom, 156 women and girls gave victim impact statements during the sentencing hearing. The media coverage of the case exposed the numerous institutions and sport governing bodies that acted complicitly and mishandled sexual abuse allegations.

Increasingly advocates characterize violence against women, as well as the term "gender-based violence," as broad terms that encompass physical, sexual, psychological, emotional, financial or social harm that are a result of historical or systemic inequality impacting female-identified persons. International human rights organizations like the United Nations (Commission on the Status of Women and the Human Rights Council) continue to report on forms of violence against women to address ongoing sexual and gender-based violence whether the context is rape as a tool of war, sexual slavery, domestic abuse, female genital mutilation or early and forced marriage. Effectively responding to gender-based violence requires addressing the multidimensional and complex circumstances impacting women's lives. Women's individual and collective experiences of violence are shaped by multiple forms of discrimination and disadvantage, which intersect with race, religion, gender identity, sexual orientation, immigrant and refugee status, disability, poverty and other markers of identity. Read from this perspective, it is impossible to understand the cause and effects of trauma as largely reducible to neurological concerns.

The Limits of the 'Neuro Revolution'

At best, it is possible to characterize the "neuro revolution" as helping to spur new discussions and discoveries. The revolution in neuroscience research has helped to anchor and advance the study of trauma as spurred by powerful neuroimaging techniques and biomedical advances, which in turn has largely emphasized the biological effects of psychological trauma (Crenshaw 2006). The concern for feminists working in the trauma sector is the "extent to which so much of our understandings of trauma are increasingly medically oriented and the assumptions that privilege *diagnostic assessments as the foundation of effective work within trauma*" (Tseris 2013, 154, emphasis added). As Herman so brilliantly outlined, responses to trauma must occur within the context of a broad social movement that works to address women's ongoing exposure to gender-based violence. This requires bearing witness, it requires activism and interventions beyond neuroscientific studies rooted in a biomedical model of trauma. Herman's message holds parallels with "neurophilosophers" and others within critical neuroscience who claim that "brainhood" is taking the place of personhood (Slaby 2010, 401). In other words, the brain-oriented approach that has driven the medicalization of trauma and has enabled work on brain-based trauma-related health issues such as hyperarousal, dissociative problems, affect dysregulation, etc., has often privileged medical knowledge over women's own narratives (Tseris 2013).

In short, we are more than our brains. Neuroscience has been endowed with legitimacy, a scientific currency, that lends itself to a privileged way of documenting and framing trauma's imprint on the brain, enabling an approach that considers the cognitive impact of violence but not its socio-political or cultural context. But what happens when systemic gender-based violence is viewed sufficiently broadly? Trauma studies is a discipline that is thick with survivor testimony (Coddington 2017). Women who have experienced sexual abuse and violence have articulated nuanced accounts of trauma. How do we resist privileging measurable, observable physiological evidence of neuropsychiatric damage over women's accounts of trauma? How do we promote a social justice framework that centres women's narratives alongside the privileged status of sophisticated imaging techniques that have become the mainstream of brain research?

A focus on neuro discourses obstructs the structural nature of our contemporary and collective exposure to violence. Moreover, it is important to acknowledge that while violence against women occurs across lines of social class, ability, race, religion, and culture, racialized women and women with disabilities experience gender-based violence often compounded by exposure to recurrent poverty and racism. As Sherene Razack (1998, 59) highlights:

> When the terrain is sexual violence, racism and sexism interlock in particularly nasty ways. These two systems operate through each other so that sexual violence, as well as women's narratives of resistance to sexual violence, cannot be understood outside of colonialism and today's ongoing racism and genocide. When women from marginalized communities speak out about sexual violence, we are naming something infinitely broader than what men do to women within our communities, an interlocking analysis that has most often been articulated by Aboriginal women.

Sexual violence, particularly against Indigenous and racialized women, is a hallmark of White settler nations such as Canada and the United States (Jiwani & Young 2006). One of the central debates in Fanon's (2005) *The Wretched of the Earth* is the relationship between trauma and colonization. He carefully highlights the planned and systemic nature of colonial trauma "locating the wounds of trauma in structured and systematic processes" (Pratt et al. 2017, 3). Indeed, everyday acts of violence against women are intimately bound with larger sociopolitical contexts including state and social responses (Pain 2014). In Canada, a National Inquiry into Missing and Murdered Indigenous Women and Girls (2019) has highlighted "the underlying social, economic, cultural, institutional, and historical causes that contribute to the ongoing violence and particular vulnerabilities of Indigenous women and girls in Canada" (www. mmiwg-ffada.ca). Violence against women and girls is a complex problem heavily mediated by relations of race, class privilege and nationality. In addition, there are social and state responses to gendered violence, such as legislation, policies and practices, that perpetuate and maintain social structures and gender inequalities that perpetuate violence. For example, the underfunding of, and limited spaces in, women's shelters, women who have precarious housing, data outlining that domestic violence still often goes unreported to police, a criminal justice system where survivors of gender-based violence do not feel supported and ineffective restraining or protective orders against male perpetrators (Sinha 2013). Fanon calls for a collective response to address the conditions that enable colonial trauma. Given the breadth and depth of personal and collective histories of trauma, there must be collective politics, there must be action. In *Black Skin, White Mask*, Fanon (channeling the revolutionary Marx) writes, "What matters is not to know the world but to change it" (2008, 17). For Fanon, understanding is not an end in itself, it must lead to change. This is also a foundation of feminist trauma work. It is at the core of SYL.

(Returning to) The Body as a Site of Trauma

My own understandings of gender-based violence and trauma have evolved over the years through my work with SYL, a free, non-contact boxing program for female-identified individuals who have experienced violence. In the 12 years of running the Toronto (Canada)-based program, over 1800 survivors of violence have participated, and we often maintain a waiting list of over 300 women seeking to access the program. SYL operates from the premise that trauma is held in people's bodies and that recovering from violence and trauma depends on experiential knowledge (Van Der Kolk 2014). In other words, when violence happens to you, the very core of your being, the safety of your own body has been violated. Recovery from trauma requires being able to feel in charge of not just your mind, as is the focus of many neurological discourses, but also of your own body, in all its visceral dimensions. Too often women do not have access to physical, body-based experiences that directly contradict the immobilization, helplessness, collapse or rage they experienced and continue to experience as part of their trauma, including head traumas (Van Der Kolk 2014). While there is no single approach to recover from trauma, women are most often directed towards talk-based therapy or pharmaceutical interventions, where they are medicated through a brain-disease model in which drugs are used to address a range of physical and psychological symptoms (insomnia, anxiety, hyperarousal, depression, nightmares, etc.). Indeed, many women in SYL are medicated (self-medicated or prescribed) and/or involved in some kind of talk-based therapy. This approach has limitations. Trauma has far-reaching implications and effective treatment and healing has to engage with the whole person, including getting in touch with their (often dissociated) bodies. To recover from violence, abuse and trauma, the body has to be experienced as a source of pleasure and comfort (Van Der Kolk 2014).

Everyday acts of violence against women have not received the levels of attention and resourcing that they merit. As feminist scholars have observed, global terrorism, which is viewed as "public, political, global and spectacular," receives much more recognition and resourcing than the everyday terrorism of intimate partner violence (Pain 2014, 532). This is notable. The least prevalent form of terrorism is given the most attention by the state while domestic violence, despite its everywhereness, is overlooked and staggeringly discounted (Pain 2014).

And yet, recent discussions of the "concussion crisis" has meant sports like boxing, football and rugby have received a great deal of media and cultural focus—which has helped to obscure one of the leading causes of head trauma: the widespread violence perpetrated by men against women. In their work on gendered violence and brain injury inside and outside of professional football, Morrison and Casper (2017) ask an important question: "What and who are we missing when we focus media and biomedical attention only on football and its injuries?" (p. 157). Their work highlights that women's traumatic brain injuries resulting from intimate partner violence are given little attention compared with the focus on professional football players or military veterans.

The brain injuries women sustain through gender-based, and in particular, intimate partner violence are vastly under-researched, under-treated and under-reported. As Morrison and Casper (2017) outline, it is not possible to address the high rates of traumatic brain injury without also addressing domestic violence and its impacts on women. For me this reveals two separate truths about gendered violence, each centered on the dialectic of trauma. First, gender-based violence, despite its everywhereness and severity, is yet to be widely understood as a source of trauma. Second, when there is recognition of gendered violence and trauma, it is too often associated with (men's) repetitive brain trauma in sport and also in war. The point I want to make in the remaining half of this paper is a simple one—and one made by many before me—that the *body* is the site of trauma. The brain is vulnerable to acute traumatic injury from gendered violence, but violence against women cannot be reduced to the injurability of the brain.

In the following section I want to return to the body as a site of trauma and consider, through the testimony of participants and my own experiences in SYL, some of the other dimensions that are part of the individual and collective experiences of trauma. Participants in SYL, whose voices are included here, discuss their relationship to their own body and the effect that boxing in a non-contact, trauma-informed boxing program had on them. While most of the research with SYL has been ethnographic and draws heavily on interviews with participants, the project received three years (2016–2019) of funding from the Public Health Agency of Canada to measure mental and physical health outcomes. Here, I draw primarily from the interview data from that study. First, however, it is important to provide some basic demographic information about the SYL boxers. Participants in SYL are female-identified and can join the program through self-referral (i.e., simply contacting the project coordinator on their own and registering for the program) or they can be referred by an outside agency (for example, a community health centre, a social worker, addictions therapist, mental health worker, etc.).

SYL participants range in age from 18 to 66 years old. While a large number of our participants deal with financial strain, housing and food security issues, it is important to recognize that a significant number of participants also hold post-secondary degrees, are business owners or work in well-paying jobs, and are financially secure. Participants are racially and ethnically diverse. Indeed, there is no typical SYL participant beyond a common experience of long-term trauma, or what is referred to as Complex Post-Traumatic Stress Disorder (C-PTSD). This means that rather than experiencing a traumatic event of time-limited duration such as a car accident or a natural disaster, participants have been exposed to multiple traumas and experienced severe psychological harm that occurred with prolonged, repeated exposure. C-PTSD, a diagnosis proposed by Judith Herman, has yet to be recognized as an official diagnosis or be included in the DSM, however, the concept is used extensively in the field of trauma. Participants in SYL include women who have witnessed and experienced domestic violence, rape and sexual assault, sex slavery and trafficking, incest, political conflict outside of the West, and long-term child physical and sexual abuse. C-PTSD has a group of symptoms that fall into three main categories: hyperarousal (where physiological arousal continues unabated); intrusion (where the trauma is revisited through flashbacks and memories as if occurring in the present); and constriction (through dissociation, a detached or altered state of consciousness). When people experience chronic trauma, it affects their brain and their body. To this point, Van der Kolk (2009, 24) explains the ways in which trauma lingers:

> What most people do not realize is that trauma is not the story of something awful that happened in the past, but the residue of imprints left behind in people's sensory and hormonal systems. Traumatized people often are terrified of the sensations of their own body.

Trauma, despite its many constant features, is not the same for everyone. It is also important to remember that while it is profoundly meaningful for participants to describe their trauma, the act of telling is not sufficient to alter the automatic physical and hormonal responses of the body that remain hypervigilant, anticipating another assault or violation in their future (Van der Kolk 2014). Here, five SYL participants briefly discuss their experience of trauma and violence. These participants have taken part in a 14-week program of SYL. Most continue to come to a grad class, a weekly slot of boxing available to any boxer who has already participated in the 14-week program. In order to protect the identity of participants, their self-selected 'boxing name' is used here. The only changes I have made to the text is some copy-editing to remove speech patterns such as "like" and "you know" as well as incomplete sentences. At no point in any interview are participants asked to discuss their traumatic experiences. In fact, as one SYL participant stated in the 2013 documentary film on SYL, "boxing is just easier than talking." However, many participants want to articulate what they are experiencing in the inner landscapes of their bodies, and in doing so, want to tell their trauma story. Isolation is a core experience of trauma and the ability to speak their experiences is also a core experience of recovery (Herman 1997). The excerpts included here challenge us to bear witness to some aspects of their present lives in light of past events.

Comet: I was really scared all the time and in a state of terror, I feel like all the time, for as long as I could really remember, since childhood I have been scared. And I got tired because now I'm 32, I got really tired of feeling so out of control in my world, in my life, and just being so depressed and miserable all the time.

Banger: I can't also speak for everyone but in my experience physical and mental abuse was a large part of my story. I've had many years where my mental health and my physical health has been terrible. I ignored my physical body for many years. And then I entered into another relationship

	that was negative and toxic and abusive. And I also didn't know how to take care of myself
Gunnz:	I was a stripper from when I was 18 until 27, so I had a pimp. A lot of my money, he took it. He basically almost killed me. But the problem was all the money and I was controlled by him. So finally I got away from him. He hit me in the head with a bat one time because he asked me if I had any respect for him and I said 'no, not anymore', because I was trying to get away from him. . . . I know my stories are kind of scattered but I'm just saying what I remember. That man would stomp on my face, give me black eyes. I'm surprised my nose looks the way it does because it has been broken once. It's straight but he got me, he broke my nose.
Nightmare Queen:	I have Multiple Concussion Syndrome. I have been smacked in the head so many times. I have complex PTSD and if somebody hits me, I literally collapse and start dissociating and am not able to respond. I have a PTSD reaction and I start dissociating so there's no way that I would even be able to defend myself . . . like I don't even know what happened that one day. I ended up on the ground, but I don't even remember getting onto the ground. . . . Dissociation is a huge symptom and I just dissociate all the time. I think especially with complex PTSD it's actually really hard to be in your body, it is intolerable.
Doc:	It has been challenging for me and I was like tripping myself up in my head . . . because of trauma I often leave my body, especially when [weeping] I don't want to do it, and I didn't want to do it because I didn't know what I was doing—like I leave my body all the time and I learned to do that really young. . . . I've been work-ing really hard at being more present in [boxing] those physically demanding moments.

Traumatic symptoms become disconnected from the episode of trauma and become embedded in and connected to everyday life. Participants like Comet share that they are walking around in their lives with an abnormal amount of fear, or as she explained "in a state of terror." She, as well as most others in the program, talk about their experiences with anxiety and depression. At a later moment in the interview Comet explains, "I'm having nightmares every night, I don't sleep. I can't have relationships; I can't be touched. It's really hard to explain it so it's nice to be able to come here." Doc and Nightmare Queen both struggle with dissociation. "Dissociation is the essence of trauma" (Van der Kolk 2014, 66). PTSD *is* dissociation, which is the experience of being detached or disconnected from your surroundings, thoughts, memories, feelings or body. Everyone experiences dissociation in some way. For example, when you are driving and get lost in thought and then can't remember ever making a turn or going past a particular location, yet you arrive at your destination. For SYL participants, dissociation enabled them to tolerate situations that were otherwise too difficult to bear. It had its purpose. Yet, now dissociation keeps them disconnected, cut off from their present ability to associate, to engage, as their experiences are still compartmentalized and they remain detached from their own body and from the world around them (Ataria 2015). Nightmare Queen and Gunnz, like a great number of SYL participants, have had skull fractures, broken noses, injured eyes and other injuries around the head, face and neck. Some have also disclosed their experiences with strangulation, which leads to anoxic or hypoxic brain injury.

Trauma-Informed Boxing

Shape Your Life is a unique program that is based on the premise that people who have experienced violence need to have *physical* experiences to restore a visceral sense of control (Van der Kolk 2014). The SYL program is trauma-informed, which means that we understand the impacts of trauma and work to ensure that SYL is welcoming and responsive to participants, whose behaviours make sense when interpreted through a trauma-informed framework. We emphasize the safety of participants and work to ensure that they have a sense of control and know they can make decisions about their bodies while at SYL. We also pay careful attention to the space of the boxing studio, including physical layout, and incorporate knowledge of trauma into the language, policies, practices and, most importantly, into the culture of SYL. These are important elements of the program and reveal that the sport of boxing—long associated with the production of debilitating head trauma—can be recreated in a new non-contact format to promote healing and a reconnection to one's body.

Here, six SYL boxers talk about the effect boxing has had on them. Their responses echo the premise that the body keeps the score.

Comet: I've been going to therapy for 7 years and needed to try something else. . . . This is the first time in my life I'm not afraid to walk alone and I was always scared of being raped. . . . And that in itself is just so good for quality of life to just be able to walk home from the bus stop and not feel like I have to hold my breath, or if I see a man I'm like, "Fuck, this is it, this is the day I die."

. . . Now I just feel much more powerful. I feel like a much more powerful person. Every time I throw a punch, it's like, there's just so much power in my body that I never knew was there and so much strength. . . . So it's nice now to be more present with myself, understand my boundaries and respect myself and just walk but feel like I'm with myself more than I ever have been. And it's really only been because of this program.

Nightmare Queen: So I've gone to lots of different things and tried different mindfulness programs and none of them have ever worked for me. I often get extremely triggered. I've had no capacity to be in my body. And so I didn't expect this, this is an unexpected side effect of Shape Your Life, but what I found is that I completely one-hundred percent was able to be here. Cause when I was doing the heavy bag, I was not thinking about anything else whatsoever. I was one-hundred percent. And so when I realized that, I was like "that was really weird." I was like one-hundred percent in my body. I was present in my body, I was like feeling my body, and I was actively doing something and so what I conclude from that is that for myself with my history of violence, it's like, what was happening when I was being assaulted was I went into submission mode and so I was still. I was not moving. So being still and being in my body is very triggering. But when I was punching the bag it was very active. And so I was in my body, in a way that was like moving, and so therefore, I was able to do it. But I didn't even think I was doing that, you know, it wasn't like I intended to do that, it just happened, you know?

Exsanguinator: So I do numerous kinds of practices in my life that are about me getting in touch with my body, inhabiting it. Yoga and meditation do other things as far as getting me in my body. But boxing is the most visceral experience I've ever had. And I'm going to get all Eastern on you in terms of the vibration—I'm talking the physical vibration, what it does and it loosens inside my body. Stuff just comes flying out, like holy crap. So stuff I didn't realize was still stuck in me has come out and some of it has been so sad. But some of it has been just amazing, there's something special about boxing, boxing is very different. . . . I tell you I leave class and my chest is stuck out 5 feet and there's this hugeness and this openness in my body

Sting: So boxing is the place that I get to come and love the snap of punching the pads and boxing is the place that I come because I need to step into a place where my body remembers that I'm strong, where my body remembers that I'm in a different place and time. And it's not just [the abuser], there's this series of traumas stored in my system from childhood. It's this domino effect all the

	way back into my childhood. And I come to boxing on Sundays to learn how to retrain that part of my body.
Tidal:	Boxing has shown me that I'm powerful because I've never actually felt this powerful. I've felt powerful in my mind sometimes and I've felt powerful in different aspects but never this much in my body, and never this comfortable in my body. I am still working on it but especially with what we've been through I think that taking back ownership of your body and making yourself feel strong is . . . there aren't enough words for that, how important that is.

What has such salience here, and what interviews have borne out over the 12 years of SYL, is that participants articulate the ways in which they are able to begin to feel safe with others, and get in touch with their dissociated bodies. Trauma studies have documented that traumatized people chronically feel unsafe in their bodies and they learn to hide from themselves (Van der Kolk 2014). At the boxing gym, participants feel that they are in charge of their bodies and have experiences that are so different than immobilization, collapse, fear, rage or any of the other imprints of trauma on the body and mind. Comet shares that she feels more grounded, more powerful, that she is more present. Nightmare Queen was not anticipating that boxing would let her be so completely engaged in a visceral experience without dissociating. The comments also reflect a tentativeness that is important to acknowledge. Learning to box does not in itself heal trauma. Participants are aware of the ways in which boxing makes them feel "in touch" with their body, that they are "retraining" what their body remembers, and that getting "in their body," as Tidal describes, involves moving through much discomfort. The project of "taking back ownership" of her body is an ongoing one.

I also want to make sure projects like SYL are not seen as simple curative interventions. There is no simple redemptive narrative here and there is no "magic bullet" or recipe for healing. The participants in SYL work hard on their recovery and encounter many ongoing challenges. Below, one boxer, Crusher, talks about how difficult it was to even experience the joys of boxing. Her experience is one that is also common, though not often discussed, particularly in body-based intervention work. For Crusher, it is quite normal to feel anxious, fearful, withdrawn, depressed, to have access to very few social supports and to be fairly heavily medicated. When she was boxing her body was engaged in a new and unfamiliar way. She would go home and then feel completely overwhelmed by having had good visceral experiences and feelings. She shared what it was like when she started coming to SYL, and how difficult it was to experience connection in all of its various forms.

Crusher:	Okay so [after SYL] I'm going to go for a walk and I'm going to cook and I'm going to just do things, not realizing that it was a lot of emotions that I was feeling that I couldn't place. That was a really

rough night. I spent about 3 hours on the phone with the Distress Centre because when I feel like that I end up hurting myself and I was not prepared for that at all. And it happened after the second [SYL class] and it happened the third, but it gradually got better and I could manage it a bit better. But it did contribute to a lot of panic coming too because if I'm going to go there I'm going to have a good time while I'm there, I'm going to work out, I'm going to feel good and then I'm going to go home and I'm going to feel like shit and I'm going to hurt myself and I'm going to do something stupid.

There is a combination of things that have happened since I started the program, my medication is a lot more managed and has made me a lot more stable, so that's helpful too. So there are definitely nights where I go home after boxing and cry but instead of taking out a knife and hurting myself I sit there and cry and I think okay why am I crying, what am I feeling, what are the things I know I have, the skills that I have to work through it and I end up writing a lot of it down.

Crusher had profoundly upsetting emotional experiences *after* attending SYL. The SYL program has a social worker that works to connect and refer participants who need additional supports, counseling or other interventions. We have also partnered with a social service agency that does direct service work with women who experience trauma. Even with this support, Crusher experienced significant trauma and was, at one point during the 14-week program, admitted to the hospital on suicide watch. She expressed to the hospital staff that SYL was an important program for her and she was given a day pass to attend a session and then returned after the SYL class to the hospital. I included her narrative here for a few reasons, one being to highlight the vastly different ways our bodies respond to trauma and recovery. The structure and workings of the brain and its neuroplasticity, in response to violence and abuse, is most certainly underlying and framing Crusher's unbearable physical and mental pain. Here I want to return to the broader argument I began with in this paper. While neuroscience can offer a better understanding of the biological reactions to trauma, and can inform treatment protocols, if we continue to treat the trauma and not its origins, we will systematically fail to address the widespread violence women experience.

The most recent cohort of participants in the Shape Your Life program walked into the gym having endured horrible events, ranging from repeated assaultive blows to the head to being raped and left for dead in a stairwell. One participant disclosed on her first day in the gym that SYL was the first program she joined after being released from the hospital after surviving 18 stab wounds from her boyfriend. The wounds on her skin, on her shoulders, hands, chest, face, and back, so clearly locate the body as her site of trauma. As Morrison and Casper (2011) note, the characteristics of traumatic injury, whether from PTSD or traumatic brain injury, "are complex and fluid; it is often unclear where one condition ends and the next begins."

Conclusion

Advances in neuroscience are leading the way in research on trauma. As Slaby (2010) pointedly argues, the emphasis on biological markers and brain scans offers a scheme of conceptualization, an explanatory pattern, where brainhood becomes the clear and concise focus. The seductive allure of neuroscience does offer much promise. Yet it also offers a pitfall—neurobiological reductionism. As Herman (2015, 263–264) has outlined:

> the history of the trauma field has shown repeatedly, increasing scientific knowledge and raising public awareness are only the first steps in efforts to end violence. Moving from awareness into social action requires a political movement strong enough to overcome pervasive denial, the passive resistance of institutional inertia, and the active resistance of those who benefit from the established order.

Until the culture of gendered violence is addressed, we will only increase our understanding of its symptoms, without ending suffering caused by injustice and oppression.

In the epilogue to the 2015 edition of *Trauma and Recovery*, Herman argues that most interpersonal violence is directed at women and children, and that most perpetrators are men well-known to their victims. Yet despite increased awareness of gendered violence, women are often not able to hold their offenders accountable, or even receive necessary support as they work on their own recovery. In Toronto, Canada, the site of the Shape Your Life program, the *Toronto Star* reported that in 2018 the wait for individual counseling at the Toronto Rape Crisis Centre—Multicultural Women Against Rape was 15 months. In addition, staff who operate the 24/7 helpline reported twice as many calls per shift from previous years (Buck 2018). In Ontario, sexual assault centres receive some provincial funding but are supplemented by donations and fundraising efforts in order to do the work of providing education, outreach, free one-one-one counseling, support groups, court accompaniments and 24-hour helplines so that when any woman over the age of 16 is assaulted, they have access to resources. Ending sexual assault and the more troubling culture of silence around sexual assault requires additional policies, resources and financial supports.

In writing this chapter, I relied heavily on Judith Herman's work, which largely focuses on the traditional psychotherapy modality of talk-based therapy. She professes that recovery from trauma and violence always begins with safety. She also argues that "safety always begins in the body" and that body-oriented therapies can play an important role. Her work on the importance of "bearing witness," along with Bessel van der Kolk's work including a focus on yoga for patients with PTSD, heavily informed the development of SYL. So, I will close by returning to the body as experienced by a SYL participant whose boxing name is "Splatter":

> I will be 43 in a couple years and in 43 years nothing else makes me feel really good about myself, like truly *inside*. And I have tried a lot of stuff and I have had therapy for years. And I know exactly what I am supposed to do with the psychologists, the psychiatrists, the social workers, or art therapists. I know what they all say and I have tried it all and this, for me, is the best thing, because it allows you to feel strong in your body and it allows you to feel like you can take care of yourself. It allows you to feel good about yourself. It allows you to feel safe inside yourself.

In this brief excerpt, Splatter touches on some aspects of the imprints of trauma on the body and the ways in which a body-oriented approach, like Shape Your Life, is an important, though overlooked, aspect of addressing violence and trauma in the lives of women.

References

Ataria, Yochai. 2015. "Sense of Ownership and Sense of Agency During Trauma." *Phenomenology and the Cognitive Sciences* 14 (1): 199–212.

Bernick, Charles and Banks, Sarah. 2013. "What boxing tells us about repetitive head trauma and the brain." *Alzheimer's Research and Therapy* 5 (3): 23–35.

Buck, Genna. 2018. "GTA Sexual Assault Crisis Centres Overwhelmed Amid #MeToo Movement." *The Toronto Star*, January 30. www.thestar.com/news/gta/2018/01/30/gta-sexual-assault-crisis-centres-overwhelmed-amid-metoo-movement.html.

Coddington, Kate. 2017. "Contagious Trauma: Reframing the Spatial Mobility of Trauma Within Advocacy Work." *Emotion, Space and Society* 24 (3): 66–73.

Crenshaw, David. 2006. "Neuroscience and Trauma Treatment: Implications for Creative Arts Therapies." In *Expressive and Creative Arts Methods for Trauma Survivors*, edited by L. Carey, 21–38. London: Jessica Kingsley Publishers.

Fanon, Frantz. 2005. *The Wretched of the Earth*. Translated by Constance Farrington. New York: Grove.

Fanon, Frantz. 2008. *Black Skin—White Masks*. Translated by Charles Lam Markmann. New York: Grove.

Fraser, Jennifer. 2014. "Claims-Making in Context: Forty Years of Canadian Feminist Activism on Violence Against Women." PhD diss., University of Ottawa.

Graham, Bryan. 2018. "'I Was Molested by Dr. Larry Nassar': How the Gymnastics Sexual Abuse Scandal Unfolded." *The Guardian*, January 27. www.theguardian.com/sport/2018/jan/27/larry-nassar-trial-gymnastics-sexual-abuse?CMP=fb_gu.

Herman, Judith. 1995. "Crime and Memory." *Bulletin of the American Academy of Psychiatry & the Law* 23 (1): 5–17.

Herman, Judith. 1997. *Trauma and Recovery: The Aftermath of Violence—From Domestic Abuse to Political Terror*. New York: Basic Books.

Herman, Judith. 2015. *Trauma and Recovery: The Aftermath of Violence—From Domestic Abuse to Political Terror,* 1R ed. New York: Basic Books.

Jiwani, Yasmin, and Mary Lynn Young. 2006. "Missing and Murdered Women: Reproducing Marginality in News Discourse." *Canadian Journal of Communication* 31 (4): 895–917.

Lundberg, George. 1986. "Boxing Should Be Banned in Civilized Countries—Round 3." *Journal of the American Medical Association* 255 (18): 2483–2485.

Martland, H.A. 1928. "Punch Drunk." *Journal of the American Medical Association* 91: 1103–1107. https://doi:10.1001/jama.1928.02700150029009.

Morrison, Daniel, and Monica Casper. 2011. "Does Traumatic Brain Injury Have a Gender?" *The Feminist Wire,* February 2. www.thefeministwire.com/2011/02/does-traumatic-brain-injury-have-a-gender/.

Morrison, Daniel, and Monica Casper. 2017. "Gender, Violence, and Brain Injury In and Out of the NFL: What counts as harm?" In *Football, Culture and Power,* edited by David J. Leonard, Kimberly B. George, and Wade Davis, 154–175. New York: Routledge.

Pain, Rachel. 2014. "Everyday Terrorism: Connecting Domestic Violence and Global Terrorism." *Progress in Human Geography* 38 (4): 531–550.

Pratt, Geraldine, Johnston, Caleb, and Banta, Vanessa. 2017. "Filipino Migrant Stories and Trauma in the Transnational Field." *Emotion, Space and Society* 29: 83–92.

Razack, Sherene. 1998. *Looking White People in the Eye: Gender, Race, and Culture in the Courtrooms and Classrooms.* Toronto: University of Toronto Press.

Sinha, Marie. 2013. "Measuring Violence Against Women: Statistical Trends 2013." *Juristat* 33 (1), https://www150.statcan.gc.ca/n1/pub/85-002-x/2013001/article/11766/11766-4-eng.htm [accessed 2 March 2019].

Skolnik-Weisberg, Deena, Frank Keil, Joshua Goodstein, Elizabeth Rawson, and Jeremy Gray. 2008. "The Seductive Allure of Neuroscience Explanations." *Journal of Cognitive Neuroscience* 20 (3): 470–477.

Slaby, Jan. 2010. "Steps Toward a Critical Neuroscience." *Phenom Enology of Cognitive Science* 9, July: 397–416.

Tseris, Emma Jane. 2013. "Trauma Theory Without Feminism? Evaluating Contemporary Understandings of Traumatized Women." *Affilia: Journal of Women and Social Work* 28 (2): 153–164.

UN General Assembly. 1979. *Convention on the Elimination of All Forms of Discrimination Against Women.* 18 December, A/RES/34/180. www.ohchr.org/Documents/ProfessionalInterest/cedaw.pdf [accessed 5 January 2018].

UN General Assembly. 1993. *Declaration on the Elimination of Violence Against Women.* December 20, A/RES/48/104, www.un.org/documents/ga/res/48/a48r104.htm [accessed 5 January 2018].

Van Der Kolk, Bessel. 2009. "Forward." In *Trauma and the Body: A Sensorimotor Approach to Psychotherapy,* edited by Claire Pain, Kekuni Minton, and Pat Ogden, xvii–xxvi. New York: W.W. Norton & Company.

Van Der Kolk, Bessel. 2014. *The Body Keeps the Score: Brain, Mind, and Body in the Healing of Trauma.* New York: Penguin Books.

Wacquant, Loic. 1995. "Pugs at Work: Bodily Capital and Bodily Labour Among Professional Boxers." *Body & Society* 1 (1): 65–93.

World Medical Association. 2017. *WMA Statement on Boxing.* 68th WMA General Assembly, Chicago, United States, www.wma.net/policies-post/wma-statement-on-boxing/ [accessed 4 January 2018].

8　The Athlete's Body and the Social Text of Suicide

Sean Brayton and Michelle T. Helstein

Over a period of four months in the spring and summer of 2011, three former professional hockey players died in unexpected ways that drew sweeping media coverage and public concern. Notable hockey "enforcers" Derek Boogaard, Wade Belak and Rick Rypien each struggled with depression and died of possible suicides, separate events that sparked widespread criticism of hockey violence and the purported dismissiveness of mental illness in the National Hockey League (NHL). The connections between contact sports, concussions and suicide were compounded in 2012 when ex-professional football player Junior Seau died of a self-inflicted gunshot wound to the chest. He was the third former National Football League (NFL) player to die of suicide in less than 18 months. Former NFL players Dave Duerson and Ray Easterling died in eerily similar ways during the winter of 2011 and the spring of 2012, respectively. While Chronic Traumatic Encephalopathy (CTE) was later found in the brains of all three athletes, which were donated for study by the families of the decedents, Duerson left a detailed request: "Please, see that my brain is given to the NFL's brain bank" (which is the Concussion Legacy Foundation at Boston University). These events represent a veritable tipping point of what critics call the "concussion crisis" in professional sports, most notably hockey and gridiron football.

In response to such events, this article takes stock of the sporting body as a site of resistance and refusal. Specifically, it examines how the suicides of former professional gridiron football players and hockey "enforcers" offer a social commentary on physical labour in late capitalism. While widespread news reports have rightly raised concern over the possible connections between contact sports, brain injuries and depression, athlete suicides can also be read collectively as a "social text." Drawing on sociological and anthropological studies of suicide as social protest, we explain how the self-destruction of the athlete's body can and should be understood less as an individual psychological aberration than as a political act, one that reflects and reacts against a specific set of socioeconomic conditions. The recent spate of athlete suicides marks a form of embodied protest that speaks to professional sport as an economic enterprise indebted to the use, abuse and "disposability" of athletic bodies as physical labour and is thereby not unrelated to the "wave of suicides" found in other industries like manufacturing and telecommunications, for instance. The political meanings of such suicides, in other words, extend well beyond the motives and intent of any individual athlete. Unlike other worker suicides, professional athletes have increasingly donated and pledged to donate their damaged brains to medical centers interested in sports neuroscience. Although the willing submission of the athlete's corpse is framed as both honourable and important in the popular press, it also taps into a wider social history of labouring bodies and "public anatomy" that may complicate the embodied protest of the suicides. To this end, we contemplate how the radical act of suicide is tempered by the act of donation that may inadvertently maintain existing relations of production in both the NFL and NHL.

Protest Suicide as Communicative Act

From 2008 to 2014, 79 workers at France Telecom (now called Orange) committed suicide, many of whom left notes attributing their actions to workplace stress. The "epidemic of suicides" at the company "coincided with the privatization and restructuring" of France Telecom whereby a workforce of *fonctionnaires* (civil servants with job security and benefits) has faced increasing psychological stress initiated by management (Waters 2014, 14). Trade union leader Patrick Ackermann explains that management had resorted to "terror tactics"—including email harassment of workers, repeated job changes and mandatory relocations—in an attempt to force the resignation of engineers, technicians and call-center operators, who would then be replaced by a more "manageable" workforce without benefits, job security and union representation. Executives at France Telecom, however, attempted to "individualize the causes of suicide, attributing it to a mental or emotional flaw in the person and disassociating it from any link to the workplace" (Ackermann cited in Waters 2014).

Just as the suicides mounted at France Telecom in May 2012, 200 workers at a Foxconn electronics plant in Wuhan, China, climbed to the factory rooftop and threatened to kill themselves if working conditions and wages did not improve (McGrath 2012). Though the incident was widely reported, protest suicide was not an isolated event at Foxconn, which produces 40% of all global electronics products (including Apple iPhones and Microsoft Xbox 360s). After 13 workers leaped to their deaths over a period of four months in 2010, management at Foxconn's Shenzhen factory installed safety nets at the dormitory rather than improve working conditions or negotiate with workers (Chan and Ngai 2010). The bosses at Foxconn attributed the suicides to personal problems and "mental health issues" of employees. As we discuss below, a similar rhetorical tactic is sometimes adopted by popular sports press in relation to the concussion-suicide connections. Conversely, activists and coworkers explained the deaths as an attempt to escape abusive management, deplorable working conditions and unfair wage policies. In short, the suicides were *social* rather than *individual*.

At France Telecom and Foxconn, in particular, suicides and a threat thereof have been used deliberately as a political tactic against management and ownership, a phenomenon that taps into a tradition of "protest suicide" in the twentieth century. From self-immolation of Buddhist monks and American Quakers in the 1960s and suicides of South Korean industrial workers to hunger strikes by British suffragettes, Irish Republican prisoners in Northern Ireland and political inmates in Turkey today, protest suicide has taken myriad forms of what Biggs calls "communicative suffering" (2004, 1). Though the cases of protest suicide are quite different, as are the political objectives, communicative suffering is one tactic within a repertoire of protest methods designed to signal both deprivation and commitment to a cause "in ways that words alone cannot" (Biggs 2004, 12). That a protester would rather suffer and die than continue to live under conditions of social, economic and spiritual dispossession is said to validate the arguments and objectives of the political movement or cause. Here "the cost of one's life is presented as of less value than the ultimate goal of changing the rules of the game" (Fierke 2012, 84). As such, Biggs notes that "suffering may help to convince bystanders that protestors have a legitimate claim of injustice" (2004, 11). In addition, communicative suffering draws attention to power asymmetries between institutions of the state and disenfranchised subjects. In South Korea, for instance, the widespread suicides of industrial workers "constitute an ultimate gesture of denial of the existing political and economic system" by "mocking" the state's purported interest in ensuring the welfare of its citizens (Kim 2008, 570). In other words, protest suicide is a "byproduct of refusing to conform to the dominant rules" in which workers experience increasing "casualization", economic uncertainty and diminished collective power (Fierke 2012, 60).

Unlike other forms of self-destruction, *protest* suicide can be distinguished by three critical traits: it involves "dying with a message, for a message, and of a message" whereby "the action invokes a reaction based on the premise that the action . . . has the potential to trigger such a reaction" (Andriolo 2006, 102). The famous self-immolation of Buddhist monk Thích Quảng Đức in 1963, for instance, was an explicit protest against the US-supported Diem regime in South Vietnam and the systemic persecution of Buddhists. Đức's protest inspired not only several followers, including the self-immolation of American Quaker Norman Morrison in 1965, but also international criticism of US involvement in the Vietnam War. Similarly, during one of the most publicized hunger strikes in Northern Ireland in 1981, where death was an accepted consequence (rather than an objective), Irish Republican inmates led by Bobby Sands sought recognition of their status as "enemy combatants" and thus prisoners of war rather than common criminals or terrorists. Support for the incarcerated Sands even lead to his successful election as a Member of Parliament less than a month before his "death fast" ended at 66 days. During earlier hunger strikes, it was once claimed that a dead inmate would "have made 100,000 Sinn Feiners out of 100,000 constitutional nationalists" or moderates (Kee cited in Biggs 2008, 8).

It is important to note that many, though certainly not all, protest suicides are conducted as a "last resort" after other methods of protest fail. To this end, Wee describes protest suicides as "extreme communicative acts" (ECAs) that "boost illocutionary force" (2004, 2162). In other words, as ECAs, protest suicides are often preceded by more conventional campaigns and activism, leaving a trail of written documentation and genealogy of struggle that is then strengthened by the death of protestors. Indeed, a genealogy of struggle is readily apparent in recent concussion litigation against the NFL alongside the suicides of former footballers (discussed later in this chapter). In each case, the political tactic is "unconventional" in the confines of struggle insofar as violence is directed towards the self rather than one's enemy.

What is perhaps most instrumental to the efficacy of protest suicide is less the intentions of the protestor or the athlete with traumatic brain injury than the social context in which the act occurs. Whereas self-sacrifice is sometimes described as an attempt to have the "last word" in a political struggle (see Billaud 2012), it is not always interpreted as such, a phenomenon that speaks to the importance of both the socially-embedded meanings of suicide and the interpreting audience. As Park explains, the meanings of self-immolation, for instance, are highly contextual; what is often dismissed as suicide and the result of mental illness in North America is often understood as "loyalty to a cause or a moral principle" in Asia (2004, 86; see also Jang 2004). So, the social context or "cultural package" often determines the meaning of the suicide irrespective of the victim's intent (Knopf 2011, 3).

This is particularly apparent in the increasing rates of combat-zone suicides amongst soldiers in the US military. Describing such soldiers as "unknowing martyrs", Knopf explains how suicides of active military personnel have been interpreted by friends and family members as signs of "anti-war protest" (2011, 2). In this case,

> though the victim him/her self may have come to their demise for entirely private, personal reasons . . . the survivors make the act visible to the general public and in so doing, the suicide becomes social commentary about the costs and horrors of warfare, and even suggests unfavorable judgment of the military establishment.
>
> (Knopf 2011,13)

Essentially, it becomes the role of the audience as "reputational entrepreneur", not the decedent or martyr, to find symbolic social resonance in an otherwise private and individual act (DeSoucey et al. 2008, 100). While the military, the state or other representatives of the established social order may attribute suicides to mental illness and "personal problems", an audience affected by the acts may assign wider social meanings to the actions of the decedent such that the suicides are reframed as symptomatic of issues beyond the confines of the individual, a trend we may find among the lawsuits against the NHL and NFL by parents of deceased athletes that suffered from concussion and head injuries.

Herein lies the importance of approaching and understanding suicides of not only political prisoners, religious figures (like Buddhist monks), industrial workers and soldiers but also professional athletes as part of a " 'cultural package' wherein the act sends a public message to the community" signalling a "mistreatment of the victim" (Knopf 2011, 3). The questions become: to what extent can suicides of former athletes be perceived as acts of protest? If the suicides are "communicative acts", what do they tell us about the industry of collision sports in North America? To explore such queries, it is imperative to outline the various connections between athletics and labour, connections that are frequently understated or "depoliticized" in mainstream sports media (Brayton et al. 2019).

The Athlete as Worker

Though the popular press often dwells on the bloated salaries of certain celebrity athletes rather than actual working conditions, sport sociologists have long known of the striking similarities between athletics and the world of work (see Beamish 2008; Brohm 1978; Gruneau 1983; Hoch 1972; Rhoden 2006; Rigauer 1981; Scott 1971, for example). Much like the factory worker of industrial capitalism, the athlete's body is disciplined, monitored and trained with great precision to maximize output and productivity. The analogy of athletes as workers is made perhaps most explicit by Brohm (1978) and Rigauer (1981), both of whom understood sport as an instrument of bourgeois rule. Brohm famously referred to sport as an "ideological apparatus" that promotes the mechanization of the body, resistance to pain (and failure to report symptoms of head injuries) and rhetoric of competition to prepare its participants for the world of wage labour. Likewise, Rigauer offered an index of similarities between athletics and labour under industrial capitalism, including the "scientification" of productivity and achievement. As athletes are reduced to numbers, records and even salaries, and as they take on highly specialized and narrow tasks, they also become vulnerable to substitution and exchange, a "principle ruthlessly applied in the field of industrial labor" (Rigauer 1981, 73). Indeed, the division of sports labour is so pervasive that athletes are not only separated by positions (defense, offense, "special teams", etc.), but they are also *reduced* to the mechanics of each task. Much as baseball pitchers and football quarterbacks are often reduced to their throwing arms and soccer stars reduced to their feet or legs, hockey enforcers and goal scorers are often reduced to their hands (for markedly different reasons, of course). While the sports "IQ" of certain athletes are often lauded—though historically along racist lines—it is only in the era of the concussion "crisis" that athletes have been overwhelmingly reduced to their brains as evidence of CTE. Incidentally, it is the separation of hand and brain, of "execution and conception", that Braverman finds especially dehumanizing about capitalism, where the labour process is "dominated . . . by speed and dexterity", repetition and routine and where "workers are reduced almost to the level of labor in its animal form" (1974, 112, 325). According to a Marxist theory of sport, then, the fragmentation of the athlete into mere appendages results in a form of estrangement from an athlete's sense of self and "species being", that is, creative capacities as unforced workers. Athletes are typically, though not exclusively, regarded as commodities and components rather than human beings, reduced almost without exception to their statistical output in televised sports highlights and fantasy sports leagues.

Much as industrial capitalism relies upon bodies disciplined and trained to act in highly specialized ways, to embrace pain, and to maximize bodily performance, so too does normative masculinity. Within the context of the North American collision sports (hockey and gridiron football) under analysis here, it is not possible to talk about labouring bodies without highlighting, even if only briefly, the ways in which this sporting labour is highly masculinized. The successful performance of normative masculinity is generally reduced to how one uses one's body (in large, forceful, aggressive and even violent ways) while simultaneously de-emphasizing or devaluing matters of the mind (fear, pain, vulnerability) (Messner 1992). Masculinity then, becomes an integral and complicit tool within sporting labour, as both labour and masculinity require that one views their athletic body as an instrument in the pursuit of productivity and invincibility, respectively and collectively. Within collision sports the masculine use of one's body is mythologized and valorized and, in so doing, serves the principles of labour as outlined by scholars like Brohm and Rigauer (Boyle 2014, 335).

This is not to suggest that athletes and workers are dominated by an industry entirely beyond their control, nor is it to situate sport as automatically oppressive. On the contrary, Rigauer recognized the radical potential of sports, noting how "athletes have genuine political interests contrary to those of the existing state" and, we might add, the sports-industrial complex (1981, 103). To illustrate, a "people's history" of US sport is rife with revolutionary figures opposed to a "white supremacist capitalist patriarchy", from Althea Gibson, Billie Jean King and Muhammad Ali to Tommy Smith, John Carlos and Curt Flood: the seven-time Golden Glove-winning Major League Baseball (MLB) player widely credited with pioneering "free agency" in the late 1960s (hooks 2004, 53). In many ways, Flood's struggles against the MLB and its reserve clause resonate with those of NFL quarterback Colin Kaepernick, whose embodied protests against racist police brutality in the US have been met by a private labour lockout of sorts by league owners (despite the quarterback's widely-acknowledged skills). Both cases illustrate not only the racist underpinnings of sports leagues organized by white owners and driven by predominantly "black muscle" but also the ways in which capital has come to dominate sport (Rhoden 2006). In leagues that often resemble modern plantation systems, neither Flood nor Kaepernick determines the location or even the possibility of their athletic employment. There are, evidently, material costs for athletic protests, especially for black athletes in a league organized and operated by predominantly white owners.

However, sports fans are often discouraged from recognizing the working-class attributes, and thus the revolutionary potential, of professional athletes, especially during the "concussion crisis." As we have argued elsewhere, during lockouts popular press typically describes athletes as "overpaid", "ungrateful" and simply unwilling to play "for the love of the game", and athletes are represented as a homogenous group wherein highly paid superstars with secure contracts symbolically stand in for all NHL and NFL athletes (Brayton et al. 2019). In addition, the physical labour of athletics may seem far removed from the daily tasks of service workers in the "post-industrial" office space (though the ubiquity of "immaterial labour" is often overstated). However, it is in the relations between owners and workers that the connections are made apparent, where there is an increasing disposability and precarity of both professional athletes and ordinary working people, often dubbed "casual labor." As the body ages and deteriorates from use and abuse on the playing field, it becomes increasingly expendable, as we are now finding explicit in relation to concussion and brain injuries. For athletes, such conditions are perhaps most visibly illustrated by damage to the body and mind and the imminent fear of losing one's (paid) position on the roster, conditions not unlike those faced by workers at France Telecom, Foxconn and an array of other workplaces in manufacturing and service industries. If suicides can be understood as part of a "repertoire of protests" at "conventional" workplaces, they can also be situated as such within the ranks of professional sports.

Athlete Suicides as Extreme Communicative Acts

Although the relations of production between labour and capital may theoretically connect professional athletes with "ordinary" workers, the acts and contexts of workplace suicides are far from identical. Factory workers at Foxconn and service workers at France Telecom, for instance, deliberately used suicide as a political tactic to draw attention to appalling working conditions in ways that are often less pronounced but still present in professional sports. Nevertheless, each suicide can be understood as a "social text" with meanings beyond a decedent's intent and embedded within precise historical moments. In other words, while the stakes, tactics and levels of political consciousness may vary across settings of suicides, they can be interpreted with a comparable sense of urgency central to working-class conflicts. In what follows, we explore how the recent suicides of former professional athletes—diverse as they may be—inform a wider discussion of "extreme communicative acts" and a "cultural package" of labour politics in the NFL and NHL.

Despite the contexts in which these deaths occurred, initial media reports and online commentary tended to individualize each act, attributing or at least connecting the deaths to the ongoing personal struggles of each player. For example, much was made of the fact that Boogaard had a history of alcohol and drug abuse, multiple attempts at rehabilitation and had been released from drug treatment just one day before his overdose (Klein 2011a). As Boogaard's father noted, "everyone said (his son) had 'off-ice' issues" and that was the focus in the days following his son's death (Branch 2012). In the case of Rypien, the focus was on his having "a big heart, a troubled mind" (Turner 2011), highlighting his ongoing struggles with depression, including his attempts to deal with these "personal problems" through two leaves of absence in his three previous NHL seasons (Klein 2011b). Similarly, it was noted with regularity that Belak had acknowledged his bouts of depression to friends and family, and confided in TSN commentator Michael Landsberg that he had been on "happy pills for 4 or 5 years" (Landsberg 2011). Reporting on Duerson highlighted a failed marriage, significant financial difficulties and his having recently filed for bankruptcy (Yerak 2011), while much was also made of Easterling's financial problems in addition to his ongoing and very public struggles with depression, insomnia and early onset Alzheimer's (Katzowitz 2012). Finally, in the case of Seau, many initial reports of his suicide noted an incident two years prior in which he had been charged with domestic violence against his girlfriend and, on the day of that arrest, driven his car off a cliff (Duke 2012). Against these individualizing tendencies, we suggest the deaths provide a political commentary that can only be comprehended in relation to the broader context of suicide as a form of bodily resistance and refusal.

For example, although former athletes have, to our knowledge, abstained from hunger strikes and self-immolation, the specific type of suicide is more than merely noteworthy. Both Duerson and Seau, for example, died of self-inflicted gunshot wounds to the chest, a relatively rare method of suicide for men (Callanan and Davis 2011). For Duerson, the method was intended to serve a wider purpose than self-destruction of the body; it was designed to preserve the brain for future scientific studies, as his suicide text message noted his wish to "see that my brain is given to the NFL's brain bank" (Herbert 2011). Incidentally, the families of both Duerson and Seau had the former athletes' brain tissue donated to the "Sports Legacy Institute" (now called the "Concussion Legacy Foundation") at Boston University School of Medicine in 2011 and the National Institute of Neurological Disorders and Stroke in 2012, respectively. Duerson's suicide suggests not only an escape from physical and mental anguish but also an attempt to "effect social change" inasmuch as "the motivation transcends the self and is concerned with altering the potential community" (Fierke 2012, 184). Since Duerson's death, the growing trend of athletes pledging to donate brain tissue posthumously has been lauded as honourable and altruistic in the popular press (see Hille 2017).

Athlete suicides can also be understood as an "extreme communicative act" that "boosts illocutionary force", including the legitimacy of former players and their legal battles in public opinion. This is especially true of Easterling, a former Atlanta Falcons safety that died by self-inflicted gunshot in 2012 after struggling with clinical depression and dementia, both of which are now identified as symptoms of brain injuries in football. Shortly before his death,

Easterling was part of a class-action lawsuit against the NFL, one that charged that the league withheld information regarding the links between brain damage and violent physical contact in the sport. To this end, Easterling's suicide can be understood as a communicative act that not only punctuates and dramatizes the grievances of the former players but also "contributes to the evocation of sympathy for the less powerful actors" (Wee 2004, 2173). After the discovery of Tau protein in his brain tissue and the subsequent diagnosis of CTE, Easterling's suicide became physical evidence of the effects of concussions and brain trauma in football. In other words, the suicide can be interpreted as part of a repertoire of protests against the NFL. As Wee points out,

> ECAs cannot simply be understood as outward expressions of actors' internal states. Rather, ECAs are in a fundamental sense performed by the actors using their bodies as sites for the public display of actions; they achieve their communicative effects in the context of a temporally unfolding political drama.
>
> (2004, 2175)

Within the "political drama" of the NFL, Easterling's suicide actually escalated the terms of the class-action lawsuit, shifting from a case of "personal injury" to one of "wrongful death" ("Federal Concussion Lawsuit" 2012). Athlete suicides, then, become "social practices" that are perhaps best understood in the present political moment defined by class conflict between owners and workers.

Evidently, the social meanings of athlete suicides depend on "reputational entrepreneurs" to "transform the bodily image into one powerful enough to break through the established social order" (DeSoucey et al. 2008, 100). Following the suicides of Duerson, Easterling, Seau and Jovan Belcher (discussed below), popular press reflected a renewed interest in league responsibility and player safety. Braiker at *The Guardian*, for instance, suggested that "Seau's death reopens debate around NFL brain injuries" (2012); Herbert at *The New York Times* insisted, after Duerson's suicide, that "the sport needs to change" (2011); Flood of *The Huffington Post* claimed that Belcher's murder of girlfriend Kasandra Perkins and his own suicide "raises questions of traumatic brain injury in the NFL" (2012); and Zirin at *The Nation* asked if the Kansas City Chiefs rather than Belcher himself "pulled the trigger" (2014). The point here is that while the suicides of Belcher, Duerson, Easterling and Seau may have been individual acts, they are collectively understood as symptomatic of unequal power relations in the NFL and the league's belated and cursory attempts to deal with brain injuries in gridiron football. Moreover, they are mobilized within an activist community seeking social and economic change, including monetary compensation. The athlete suicides may have been "expressive for the individual" but are "given a primarily instrumental focus by those within the cause" (Jorgensen-Earp 1987, 85). The suicides, then, become social commentaries rather than individual psychological anomalies, but only through the deliberate efforts of activists, litigators and certain sports writers, all of which perform the role of "reputational entrepreneur."

Similar figures have emerged to mobilize the apparent suicides of former "enforcers" in the NHL. Much like the families of deceased soldiers, the parents of Boogaard, for example, are currently suing both the players association and the NHL for their roles in failing to file grievances with specific teams and failing to treat Boogaard's drug addictions that apparently resulted from his brain injuries while playing. Incidentally, Boogaard, Rypien and Belak all struggled with depression, which is increasingly reported among former hockey "enforcers," It is, in other words, the ways in which the apparent and confirmed suicides of Boogaard, Belak, and Rypien are understood, interpreted and actuated through litigation against sports leagues and teams that constitutes some of the political effects of "protest suicide." This is revealed by the myriad lawsuits against the NHL and NFL following the (apparent and confirmed) suicides of the leagues' workers. According to the "NFL Concussion Lawsuits" website, there are more than 4,800 former players as plaintiffs in more than 242 concussion-related lawsuits against the NFL. And in the NHL, 10 former players filed a class-action lawsuit in November 2013 against the league for its role in allegedly concealing information about head trauma. By November 2015 the number of plaintiffs grew to 92 (and at the time of this writing, is at 105).

Joining the list of plaintiffs are the parents of former NHL player Steve Montador, who suffered depression throughout his early retirement and died in 2015 of an apparent suicide by drug overdose. Montador's parents claim their son's concussion problems—which would be diagnosed posthumously as CTE—were inadequately managed by team trainers and physicians and that Montador "felt he was pressured to play, thereby keeping his place in the lineup, when he was still suffering from the effects of a concussion and was not healthy enough to play" (Campbell 2015). Although the NHL has denied any connections between Montador's death and his sports career, and sports writers often insist on the player's personal responsibility for participating in dangerous activities as well as the "generous" compensation, the suicide draws conspicuous attention to the often-unacknowledged effects of "forced labour" in professional sports. A similar lawsuit was recently filed by Cheryl Shepherd, the mother of Kansas City Chiefs linebacker Jovan Belcher, who murdered his girlfriend, then himself, with a handgun in front of coaches in December 2012. The lawsuit against the Kansas City Chiefs is for wrongful death; the plaintiff claims that Chiefs' medical staff controlled every aspect of Belcher's physical health but overlooked his mental health. Moreover, the lawsuit charges that "the Defendants disregarded evidence of impairment and fostered an environment where the Decedent was required to play through his injuries and become exposed to further neurological harm" (Kalaf 2014, para. 5). As Knopf contends, "the suicide becomes a symbol for these problems, making the private death public and the personal suicide one of protest" (2011, 15). The parents of Montador and Belcher, then, have situated the suicides of their athlete sons "in the service of a public concern" (Knopf 2011, 12).

What all of this fallout suggests is that while athlete suicides may be attributed by some to individual problems or psychological anomalies rooted solely in the player's damaged brain, the suicides are increasingly and importantly seen as collective, political and communicative—that is, as intimately related to working conditions and (mis)treatment by employers. Although the suicides of former professional athletes are often connected to a biogenic model of understanding mental illness and depression—one that is heavily criticized by many social scientists—the discussion is regularly redirected towards social structures, that is, working conditions on the playing fields and arenas. Herein lies a relatively nuanced narrative of mental health, one that traces suicide and depression to the body and biology, which is adversely affected by unsafe social conditions engendered by the economic interests of owners and managers. The suicidal and mentally-ill (former) worker is not a psychological oddity—as the management of France Telecom, Foxconn and perhaps the NHL and NFL would have us believe—but rather a product of their own working conditions. As a result, the act of self-termination may serve as a rather acute commentary less on mental health in North America than on the dangers of physical toil and collective pressure to play while seriously injured.

The significance of the sporting body is noteworthy here. At its intersections with labour, late capitalism and masculinity, the athlete's body is the most important tool in expressions of productivity (roster spots, wins, paychecks, dominance, respect). In life, athletes must guard against acknowledgement of bodily weakness or vulnerability, but in death by suicide the athlete destroys the very embodiment of invincible productivity. The suicide conveys a level of agency through and over the body that the athlete lacked in life given the conditions of their sporting labour. As such, the suicide communicates in death what the athlete could perhaps not in life. This is particularly telling in the case of Duerson, wherein the body was purposefully destroyed while the brain was spared, an agentive act which takes back control of the body but donates/spares the brain in an attempt to provide evidence of the critique being communicated through death. It is not surprising then, that many families have willingly donated brain tissue of the "dead worker" to various medical institutions for scientific study, a practice with a rather thorny reputation in working-class history that has yet to be addressed in relation to athletes and brain damage.

Brain Donation and a Political Economy of the Athlete's Corpse

Since 2008, the Concussion Legacy Foundation has secured nearly 1,500 pledges from former athletes and military veterans to become brain donors (Hille 2017). These pledges add to the existing 425 brains from deceased athletes already kept at Boston University, which is one site amongst many others devoted to researching sports and brain injuries. It is necessary to explore the practice of brain donation by positioning it alongside a more complicated social history of labouring bodies, public anatomy and class struggle to ask questions about "productivity" and the extraction of value from working bodies, dead and alive. While we detail this argument more specifically elsewhere (Brayton and Helstein 2018), it is vital to address it briefly here to necessarily temper the idea that somehow science and knowing more will alone change the relations of production within professional sport.

The struggle over dead labouring bodies—especially those of executed felons—was particularly prominent, for instance, in eighteenth century England. As Linebaugh explains, "the history of the London poor and the history of English science intersect" during the 1700s such that "a precondition of progress in anatomy depended upon the ability of the surgeons to snatch the bodies of those hanged" (1976, 69). Rejecting the surgeons' orders for dissection and public anatomy—which doubled as a deterrent by the state—the working poor often incited riots to reclaim the body of the executed (Linebaugh 1976). While there were logical, spiritual and superstitious reasons for doing so, the act also marked a rejection of the corpse's commodification (Linebaugh 1976). As McNally suggests, "In burying it intact, [the working classes] claimed a moral victory over the dismembering powers of capital" (2011, 23). It was, after all, an era in which the corpse became "a commodity with all the attributes of a property" to be "bought and sold" and "owned privately" (Linebaugh 1976, 72). To this end, "the corpse-economy . . . became a symbolic register for all that was objectionable about emergent capitalism, of its demonic drive to exploit human life and labor, of its propensity to humiliate and demean in both life and death" (McNally 2011, 58–59). Reclaiming the corpse, then, was a deliberate negation of capital's demand for "productivity."

In contrast, voluntary brain donation celebrates a return to "productivity." What we find, then, is a rather circuitous narrative of "productivity"; the athlete passes from a stage of "value" on the playing field to a stage of retirement where the body is "decommissioned" as no longer "productive" for team owners and is thereby devoid of "value." This is illustrated by the alleged inadequacies of players associations and leagues to monitor and support the health, well-being and life transition of recently retired athletes (Jhaveri 2015). Following death and organ donation, however, the body returns to a stage of "productivity" in which damaged organs become the raw materials for the development of scientific knowledge, which is presumably used to protect other athletes. Wherein for the working poor of the eighteenth century, saving the body from the surgeon's dissection scalpel marked a rejection of the corpse's commodification, we argue that brain donation may in fact inadvertently support the same sports-industrial complex that is otherwise and effectively exposed by the suicides themselves.

Interestingly, the pledge of donation among current athletes is often pitched as honourable if not obvious and has been described as a "profound action . . . to help ensure the safety and welfare" of current and future athletes (Morey, cited in Hille 2017). Whereas several NFL players pledged to donate their brains in honour of former teammates, others perceived the act of donation as commonsensical (Hille 2017). While the pledge may seem beneficial to both players and leagues, the extent to which player safety automatically improves through brain donation is highly questionable. Worker safety, for example, is typically understood and appreciated in a lexicon of "assets", "investments" and "liabilities" favoured by owners and managers whereby the player is simply a (compliant or obstinate) worker whose potential value rests in the present and immediate future, not during retirement when advanced symptoms of brain trauma routinely appear (see Arai et al. 2014; Carlson and Donavan 2013; Kedar-Levy and Bar-Eli 2008; Smith 2013). While it is difficult to dispute the recent findings of neuroscience in sports and the goodwill of former athletes offering their bodies to science, the donation of the concussed brain is still embedded within the "dismembering powers of capital." Much as the labouring body is often reduced to "fodder for industry" (i.e., the NHL or NFL), it is posthumously fodder for the "surgeon's scalpel", only now the public anatomy assumes less grotesque and more digitized forms (i.e., positron emission tomography or "PET" scan) but is no less available for audience scrutiny (McNally 2011, 57).

As honourable and heroic as it may be, the knowledge gained is still mobilized within professional sport by medical staff accountable to owners, and regardless of awareness, players are still in positions of precarity wherein choosing to acknowledge and follow protocol may cost them their position on the roster. Team physicians and trainers are embedded within a medical establishment and set of disciplinary practices that produce pressure to overlook player safety by acquiescing to the interests of their employers, that is, the interests of capital (Dasgupta and O'Connor 2013). In December 2017, for example, the Seattle Seahawks were fined a relatively paltry $100,000 for violating concussion protocol after quarterback Russell Wilson was sidelined by a hit from an Arizona Cardinals player, but returned to play without proper examination. Here the immediate value of a team's quarterback is clearly anathema to the long-term interests of player safety and concussion protocol. Similarly, the central claim of Shepherd's lawsuit against the Kansas City Chiefs is that coaches and team trainers pressured her son to play while concussed and injured. As Zirin remarks, it is possible that trainers, physicians and coaches used their "'class leverage' to compel Belcher to wreck his own brain" (2014). Here it is difficult to fathom how such indiscretions would be eliminated through increased brain donations.

Hypothetically, however, the increasing visibility of the public anatomy of athletes' brains and the presence of CTE could further diminish already-dwindling public support of collision sports, eventually draining the labour pool of potential players. Grier and Cowen outline the prospective fallout, wherein as "technological solutions (new helmets, pads) are tried and they fail", fewer will be willing to see the game as worth it, feeder leagues will diminish, and "the socioeconomic picture of a football player becomes more homogenous: racialized, poor, weak home life, poorly educated (2012). Of course, this might not sound the death knell of football entirely. As Zirin has pointed out, many NFL players, for instance, already emerge from racialized communities and from a lower socioeconomic background, often without graduating from college or university (2011). Nevertheless, alongside a growing number of former NFL players that have sworn to prevent their children from playing football—including Bo Jackson, Brett Favre, Arian Foster and Drew Brees—support for youth football is increasingly dubious because of what we now know of the sport and brain injuries; a recent article in *GQ* magazine asks, "What kind of father lets his son play football" (Zaleski 2017)? In the event of Grier and Cowen's scenario, then, the NFL would rely on "much lower talent levels, less training, and probably greater player representation from poorer countries, where the demand for money is higher and the demand for safety is lower" (2012). In other words, collision sports would rely more heavily on outsourced labour, which is typically sought in other industries for its compliance with low wages and poor working conditions.

As some sports commentators have concluded, while gridiron football and hockey may become incrementally "safer" because of medical advancements, the sports (and professions) remain inherently and overwhelmingly dangerous (Grier and Cowen 2012). According to Seattle Seahawks Pro Bowl cornerback Richard Sherman, the NFL's recent attention to concussion protocol—including escalated fines for illegal hitting, increased on-field medical staff and the league's donations to neuroscientific research—is merely about "optics" and "public opinion" rather than player safety since "there are still players going back into the game after head injuries and after huge collisions" (cited in Holmes 2017). Sherman insists that measures such as fines and penalties merely punish players (as workers) rather than improve the safety of the game. Much of this is a result of the current framing of problems in collision sports as a "concussion crisis" (rather than an "existential" one), which allows the NFL and other leagues "to treat the crisis as a function of improper tackling, of inadequate rules, of insufficient education, of the behavior of an isolated group of bad actors" (Mahler 2012). A similar narrative exists in the NHL where "aggressive" players are tagged as "a huge part of the problem" (Jhaveri 2015). In other words, the concussion "crisis" locates the problem in "how the game is played, not from the game itself": an "inherently violent" sport where even "unremarkable plays can eventually add up to permanent brain damage" (Mahler 2012).

Conclusion

"Given its self-destructive finality" protest suicide is "utter[ly] dependent on others to continue the process sparked by the departure of its initiator" (Andriolo 2006, 107). That is, in any act of protest suicide "how the death is interpreted [and] memorialized" by the living recreates and determines the expression of the act. The difficulty here is that the powerful can and often do quickly recreate the act within the framework of individual (in)stability and (ir)respsonsibilty. We have certainly seen this within reactions to athlete suicides in the NHL and NFL. As is common with protest suicide, the successful individualizing of the suicide act diminishes its ability to unsettle the conditions in which it occurred.

However, as the sociological literature points out, the queue of corpses disrupts the ability to ignore the political message. One Foxconn or France Telecom worker who jumps to their death may be easily dismissed as mentally unstable, but the collection of jumpers increasingly becomes more difficult to frame as a problem or weakness of an individual. This is also true of athlete suicides which occurred during heightened debates over player safety and brain injury as well as labour lockouts in the NFL and NHL, enabling the suicides to "boost illocutionary force." More than psychological aberrations, the suicides of professional athletes provide insight into the (un)sustainability of dominant sports industries. Noticing the collective conditions of these suicides requires us to make questions of labour central to our understanding of the suicide acts. It seems the subject of suicide has never been more deeply embedded in working conditions, expendability and the dehumanizing tendencies of late capitalism as in the "age of austerity", as illustrated by collective suicides of engineers, technicians and telephone operators at France Telecom, factory workers at Foxconn, farmers in India and former professional athletes of collision sports in North America (Breslow 2014; Chakrobortty 2013; Umar 2015; Waters 2014). Repositioning the suicides in this way, highlights socialist-inspired critiques of sport as a handmaiden of capitalism, positing athletic bodies as "productive" (through the extraction of value) both in life, and now, in death.

Thus, while the athletes may or may not have designed their suicides as statements of protest against the use, abuse and "disposability" of athletic bodies as physical labour, and may or may not have had personal struggles, their actions can and should be understood within these conditions and norms in which their suicides occurred. That is, rather than dismissing each suicide as an act which says something about the characteristics of the individual, as those now left behind to memorialize the act, we have an obligation to acknowledge and extend the expression of the act as social, collective, political and communicative.

References

Andriolo, Karin. 2006. "The Twice-killed: Imagining Protest Suicide." *American Anthropologist* 108 (1): 100–113.

Arai, Akiko, Yong-Jae Ko, and Stephen Ross. 2014. "Branding Athletes: Exploration and Conceptualization of Athlete Brand Image." *Sport Management Review* 17 (2): 97–106.

Bairner, Alan. 2007. "Back to Basics: Class, Social Theory, and Sport." *Sociology of Sport Journal* 24 (1): 20–36.

Beamish, Rob. 2008. "Marxism, Alienation and Coubertin's Olympic Project." In *Marxism, Cultural Studies and Sport*, edited by Ben Carrington, and Ian McDonald, 88–105. New York and London: Routledge.

Biggs, Michael. 2004. "When Costs are Beneficial; Protest as Communicative Suffering." *Paper Presented at the Meeting of the American Sociological Association.* San Francisco, CA.

Biggs, Michael. 2005. "Dying Without Killing: Self-immolations, 1963–2002." In *Making Sense of Suicide Missions*, edited by Diego Gambetta, 173–208. Oxford: Oxford University Press.

Biggs, Michael. 2008. "Dying for a Cause—Alone?" *Contexts* 7 (1): 22–27.

Billaud, Julie. 2012. "Suicidal Performances: Voicing Discontent in a Girls' Dormitory in Kabul." *Cultural Medical Psychiatry* 36: 264–285.

Boyle, Ellexis. 2014. "Requiem for a "tough guy": Representing Hockey Labor Violence and Masculinity in Goon." *Sociology of Sport Journal* 31: 327–348.

Braiker, Brian. 2012. "Junior Seau's Death Reopens Debate Around NFL Brain Injuries." *The Guardian*, May 3. www.theguardian.com/sport/us-news-blog/2012/may/03/junior-seau-nfl-brain-injuries.

Branch, John. 2012. "In Hockey Enforcer's Descent, a Flood of Prescription Drugs." *New York Times*, June 4. www.nytimes.com/2012/06/04/sports/hockey/in-hockey-enforcers-descent-a-flood-of-prescription-drugs.html

Braverman, Harry. 1974. *Labor and Monopoly Capital: The Degradation of Work in the Twentieth Century*. New York: Monthly Review Press.

Brayton, Sean and Michelle T. Helstein. 2018. "Brain Donations and a Political Economy of the Athlete's Corpse." *Presentation at the annual meeting of the North American Society for the Sociology of Sport*. Vancouver: Canada.

Brayton, Sean, Michelle Helstein, Mike Ramsey, and Nicholas Rickards. 2019. "Exploring the Missing Link Between the Concussion "crisis" and Labor Politics in Professional Sports." *Communication and Sport* 7 (1), 110–131.

Breslow, Jason. 2014. "76 of 79 Deceased NFL Players Found to Have Brain Disease." *PBS Frontline*, September 30. www.pbs.org/wgbh/frontline/article/76-of-79-deceased-nfl-players-found-to-have-brain-disease/.

Brohm, Jean-Marie. 1978. *Sport: A Prison of Measured Time*. Translated by Ian Fraser. London: Ink Links.

Callanan, Valerie J., and Mark S. Davis. 2011. "Gender and Suicide Method: Do Women Avoid Facial Disfiguration?" *Sex Roles* 65: 867–879.

Campbell, Ken. 2015. May 12. "Steve Montador Had Extensive CTE, but Mystery Surrounds Lawsuit and Cause of Death." *The Hockey News*, May 12. www.thehockeynews.com/news/article/steve-montador-had-extensive-cte-but-mystery-surrounds-lawsuit-and-cause-of-death

Carlson, Brad D., and Todd Donavan. 2013. "Human Brands in Sport: Athlete Brand Personality and Identification." *Journal of Sport Management* 27 (3): 193–206.

Chakrabortty, Aditya. 2013. "The Woman Who Nearly Died Making Your iPad." *The Guardian*, August 5. www.theguardian.com/commentisfree/2013/aug/05/woman-nearly-died-making-ipad.

Chan, Jenny, and Pun Ngai. 2010. "Suicide as Protest for the New Generation of Chinese Migrant Workers: Foxconn, Global Capital, and the State." *The Asia-Pacific Journal* 8 (37): 1–33.

Dasgupta, Ishan, and Dan O'Connor. 2013. "From Sports Ethics to Labor Relations." *The American Journal of Bioethics* 13 (10): 17–18.

DeSoucey, Michaela, Jo-Ellen Pozner, Corey Fields, Kerry Dobransky, and Gary Alan Fine. 2008. "Memory and Sacrifice: Am Embodied Theory of Martyrdom." *Cultural Sociology* 2 (1): 99–121.

Duke, Alan. 2012. "Former NFL Player Junior Seau Dead." *CNN*, May 3. www.cnn.com/2012/05/02/sport/nfl-seau-dead/index.html

Durkheim, Emile. 1952. *Suicide: A Study in Sociology*. London: Routledge.

Fassin, Didier. 2011. "The Trace: Violence, Truth, and the Politics of the Body." *Social Research* 78 (2): 281–298.

"Federal Concussion Lawsuit Changes with Death of Ray Easterling." *NFL.com*, April 23, 2012. www.nfl.com/news/story/09000d5d828867e0/article/federal-concussion-lawsuit-changes-with-death-of-ray-easterling

Fierke, K.M. 2012. *Political Self-sacrifice: Agency, Body and Emotion in International Relations*. Cambridge: Cambridge University Press.

Flood, Derek. 2012. "Jovan Belcher's Murder-suicide Raises Questions of Traumatic Brain Injury in the NFL." *The Huffington Post*, December 3. www.huffingtonpost.com/derek-flood/jovan-belchers-murdersuic_b_2229009.html

Giulianotti, Richard. 2005. *Sport: A Critical Sociology*. Cambridge: Polity Press.

Grier, Kevin, and Tyler Cowen. 2012. "What Would the End of Football Look Like?" *Grantland*, February 13. http://grantland.com/features/cte-concussion-crisis-economic-look-end-football/

Gruneau, Riachrd. 1983. *Class, Sports and Social Development*. Amherst: University of Massachusetts Press.

Herbert, Bob. 2011. "The Sport Needs to Change." *The New York Times*, March 15. www.nytimes.com/2011/03/15/opinion/15herbert.html

Hille, Bob. 2017. "30 Former NFL Players Donate Brains to CTE Research, Foundation Says." *The Sporting News*, February 3. www.sportingnews.com/nfl/news/30-former-nfl-players-donate-brains-to-cte-research-foundation-says/dtinsms0ww6q1mo1pqlc7kujr

Hoch, Paul. 1972. *Rip Off the Big Game*. New York: Anchor Books.

Holmes, Jack. 2017. "Richard Sherman on NFL protests, Trump, and this Particular Media Moment." *Esquire*, December 8. www.esquire.com/sports/a14323331/richard-sherman-nfl-protests-kaepernick-trump/

hooks, bell. 2004. *We Real Cool: Black Men and Masculinity*. London and New York: Routledge.

Jang, Sang-Hwan. 2004. "Continuing Suicide Among Laborers in Korea." *Labor History* 45 (3): 271–297.

Jhaveri, Hemal. 2015. "Daniel Carcillo Opens Up About Steve Montador's Death: 'I Was Inconsolable'." *USA Today*, April 22. http://ftw.usatoday.com/2015/04/daniel-carcillio-steve-montador-concussions

Jorgensen-Earp, Cheryl R. 1987. "'Toys of Desperation': Suicide as Protest Rhetoric." *Southern Speech Communication Journal* 53 (1): 80–96.

Kalaf, Samer. 2014. "Jovan Belcher's Mother Files Wrongful Death Suit Against Chiefs." *Deadspin*, January 2. https://deadspin.com/jovan-belchers-mother-files-wrongful-death-lawsuit-aga-1493654475

Katzowitz, Josh. 2012. "Before Committing Suicide, Ray Easterling Reached Out to Harry Carson for Help." *CBS Sports*, June 10. www.cbssports.com/nfl/news/before-committing-suicide-ray-easterling-reached-out-to-harry-carson-for-help/

Kedar-Levy, Haim, and M. Michael Bar-Eli. 2008. "The Valuation of Athletes as Risky: A Theoretical Model." *Journal of Sport Management* 22 (1): 50–81.

Kim, Hyojoung. 2008. "Micromobilization and Suicide Protest in South Korea, 1970–2004." *Social Research* 75 (2): 543–578.

Klein, Jeff Z. 2011a. "Boogaard Died from Alcohol and Drug Mix." *New York Times*, May 20. www.nytimes.com/2011/05/21/sports/hockey/boogaard-died-from-mix-of-alcohol-and-oxycodone.html

Klein, Jeff Z. 2011b. "Player's Death Follows Bouts of Depression." *New York Times*, August 16. www.nytimes.com/2011/08/17/sports/hockey/rypiens-death-follows-bouts-of-depression.html

Knopf, Christina. 2011. "Unknowing Martyrs in the Anti-war Cause: The Creation of Protest Statements Through Combat-zone Suicides." *Paper Presented at the Meeting of the American Sociological Association.* Las Vegas, NV.

Landsberg, Michael. 2011. "Depression—and My Friend, Wade Belak." *TSN Hockey*, September 13. www.tsn.ca/depression-and-my-friend-wade-belak-from-sept-13-2011-1.340782

Linebaugh, Peter. 1976. "The Tyburn Riot Against the Surgeons." In *Albion's Fatal Tree: Crime and Society in Eighteenth Century England*, edited by Douglas Hay, Peter Linebaugh, John Rule, E.P. Thompson, and Cal Winslow, 65–117. New York: Pantheon.

Mahler, Jonathan. 2012. "Why the NFL's 'Concussion Crisis' isn't Really a Concussion Crisis." *Deadspin*, December 7. https://deadspin.com/5966319/why-the-nfls-concussion-crisis-isnt-really-a-concussion-crisis

McGrath, Ben. 2012. "China: Two Hundred Foxconn Workers Threaten Suicide." *World Socialist Website*, May 12. www.wsws.org/en/articles/2012/05/foxn-m12.html

McNally, David. 2011. *Monsters of the Market: Zombies, Vampires and Global Capitalism.* Leiden and Boston: Haymarket.

Messner, Michael. 1992. *Power at Play: Sports and the Problem of Masculinity.* Boston: Beacon Press.

Park, B.C. Ben. 2004. "Sociopolitical Contexts of Self-immolation in Vietnam and South Korea." *Archives of Suicide Research* 8: 81–97.

Pratt, Geraldine, Caleb Johnston, and Vanessa Banta. 2017. "Filipino Migrant Stories and Trauma in the Transnational Field." *Emotion, Space and Society* 29: 83–92.

Rhoden, William. 2006. *Forty Million Dollar Slaves.* New York: Crown.

Rigauer, Bero. 1981. *Sport and Work.* Translated by Allan Guttman. New York: Columbia University Press.

Scott, Jack. 1971. *The Athletic Revolution.* New York: Free Press.

Smith, Rodney K. 2013. "Solving the Concussion Problem And Saving Professional Football." *Thomas Jefferson Law Review* 35 (2): 127–191.

Stack, Steven. 2004. "Emile Durkheim and the Altruistic Suicide." *Archives of Suicide Research* 8: 9–22.

Turner, Randy. 2011. "A Big Heart, a Troubled Mind: Rick Rypien." *Winnipeg Free Press*, August 10. www.winnipegfreepress.com/opinion/fyi/a-big-heart-a-troubled-mind 131379493.html

Umar, Baba. 2015. "India's Shocking Farmer Suicides." *Al Jazeera*, May 18. www.aljazeera.com/indepth/features/2015/05/india-shocking-farmer-suicide-epidemic-150513121717412.html.

Waters, Sarah. 2014. "Capitalism's Victims." *Jacobin*, December 13. www. jacobinmag.com/2014/11/capitalisms-victims/.

Wee, Lionel. 2004. "'Extreme Communicative Acts' and the Boosting of Illocutionary Force." *Journal of Pragmatics* 36: 2161–2178.

Yeak, Becky. 2011. "Duerson Had Filed for Personal Bankruptcy." *Chicago Tribune*, February 22. http://articles.chicagotribune.com/2011-02-22/sports/ct-spt-0222-duerson-bankruptcy-20110222_1_alicia-duerson-freezer-supplier-bankruptcy-filing

Zaleski, Luke. 2017. "What Kind of Father Lets His Son Play Football?" *GQ*, August 16. www.gq.com/story/should-i-let-my-son-play-football

Zirin, Dave. 2011. "Against All Odds: NFL Players Association Emerges from Lockout as Bruised, Battered Victors." *The Nation*, July 25. www.thenation.com/article/against-all-odds-nfl-players-association-emerges-lockout-bruised-battered-victors/

Zirin, Dave. 2014. "Jovan Belcher's Murder-suicide: Did the Kansas City Chiefs Pull the Trigger?" *The Nation*, January 6. www.thenation.com/article/jovan-belchers-murder-suicide-did-kansas-city-chiefs-pull-trigger/

9   Brain Politics

Gendered Difference and Traumatic Brain Injury in Sport

Kathryn Henne

Introduction

Media coverage of high-profile lawsuits involving professional sport leagues in North America has helped to raise awareness of the long-term and embodied effects of traumatic brain injury (TBI). While these developments mark a shift in public consciousness about concussions in sport, questions remain about underlying relationships between TBI, concussion, and long-term degenerative brain disease, and terminology is often confusing and imprecise (see Sharpe and Jenkins 2015; Tagge et al. 2018). Further, public narratives about concussions rarely acknowledge that the vast majority of people affected by TBI are not male athletes in collision sports, but rather, children and the elderly—as falls (48%) are the primary cause of TBI in the United States (Centers for Disease Control and Prevention 2019).

In response to the popular emphasis on men's collision sports, this chapter examines gendered contours of concussion and TBI through a focus on how U.S.-based advocates and experts tend to frame them in relation to women, considering their implications for understandings of TBI among participants in women's sports. These concerns emerge against a wider push to highlight how research, resources, and rhetoric disproportionately concentrate on TBI in men to the detriment of women's health and well-being. A range of topics fall within advocacy around TBI among women and, in turn, the scope of this chapter: the underrepresentation of women in TBI clinical trials, the exclusion of female subjects from pre-clinical trials, speculations that strength differentials between male and female athletes affect TBI occurrence rates, and concerns regarding the quality and amount of data on TBI in women's sports.

Here, I consider how knowledge production and advocacy efforts around TBI contribute to the social construction of female athletes, their bodies, and their brains. My aim is not simply to analyze gendered issues related to concussions among women, but to bring feminist concerns in dialogue with attempts to unpack how interpretations of science inform framings of concussion crises in sport (e.g., Ventresca 2019)—a concern this is especially important given the rise of evidence-based governance in sport and beyond (Palmer 2013; Merry and Coutin 2014; Henne and Pape 2018). In particular, scrutinizing efforts to capture and explain women's experiences of TBI in popular, regulatory, and scientific narratives illuminates complications between notions of sex and gender.

While "the treatment of the biological and social as separate spheres has been both commonplace and complicated," many feminist inquiries have shifted to address "the co-constitution of nature and culture" (Pitts-Taylor 2016, 10). Feminists have come to acknowledge—and in fact, interrogate—the category of "sex" as not being limited to the domain of biology. "Gender" is also not confined to the social; rather, sex/gender are inextricably linked in ways that have embodied implications (Fausto-Sterling 2005).[1] As Banu Subramaniam (2009, 956) explains, "[c]ulture is literally written on the body," and it is important to attend to how the "body seems much too complex to reduce to easy questions of biology versus socialization" (969). Rather than pose questions whether or not and how "nature" or "nurture" affects TBI among women in sport, I ask: how do sex/gender, science, and sport contribute to the construction of TBI in female athletes?

Feminist research concerned with neuroscience and the brain offers a starting point for this inquiry (e.g., Dussauge and Kaiser 2012; Jordan-Young 2011; Pitts-Taylor 2016; Roy 2016). Although scholars have troubled sex/gender relationships for some time, Isabelle Dussauge and Anelis Kaiser (2012, 212) highlight the comparative "invisibility of gender—and other power orderings usually addressed in feminist studies, such as sexuality or race—" among "critical engagements with the 'neuro' in interdisciplinary settings." In response, they point to the shared belief among many scholars "that what culturally passes as sex is indeed already gender. In the neurosciences too, it is becoming increasingly evident that the biological and social components of a gendered brain function or structure cannot be separated" (Dussauge and Kaiser 2012, 212). Attempts to separate sex from gender misconstrue the co-constitutive nature of bodies, the multiplicity of which is well documented. According to Victoria Pitts-Taylor (2016, 9), "there is not *a* body as such, but rather bod*ies*, which are historically situated, socially stratified, and differentially experienced." In her own work, Pitts-Taylor (2016, 1) has interrogated the meanings, discourses, and biology of bodies *with* brains, illustrating how shifting understandings of the brain inform two emergent concerns: that the brain is "conceived of as the biological ground for the self and social life" and is "understood as itself a product of sociality, built through experience and open to transformation." Taken together, these critical insights into bodies and brains offer us at least three key observations: (1) that biology and society are not dichotomies, (2) that sex/gender are not distinct, and (3) that the brain is embodied and social—and thus gendered. How, then, might these observations come to bear on questions of TBI and bodies with injured brains, especially when those bodies are identified as women?

As discussed in the pages that follow, narratives around sports concussions among women are not simply modes through which their bodies become understood by different actors; they aid in constituting injury among female athletes as distinct from those experienced by male athletes. In doing so, they minimize the multiplicity of bodies in favor of more essentialized gender constructs along binary lines of difference. Scrutinizing how sport-related concussion becomes gendered in this way enables us to see how TBI in women becomes *enacted*—that is, as Annemarie Mol (2003) explains, the collaborative dynamics that enable a thing to come into being. It also offers a contemporary example of how ideology, science, and sex/gender converge in relation to women's bodies. As work by feminist sport scholars, such as Jennifer Hargreaves (1994) and Patricia Vertinsky (1987), attests, nineteenth and twentieth century ideologies and medical explanations about women's bodies have "contributed substantially to a deepening stereotyping of women as both the weaker and a periodically weakened sex," which are myths that "female athletes and feminists have worked hard to dispel" (Vertinsky 1987, 8). Even though women's sport is more widely accepted today, advocacy and research often convey tacit assumptions regarding the inferiority of women's bodies, including subscriptions to longstanding narratives that recast sport-specific issues as "problems" associated with being female.

This analysis examines how emergent approaches to understanding TBI in women reveal a continuation of reductionist framings articulated through the discourse of female physiology while also attending to shifting norms that span sport and biomedical science. Specifically, it offers insights into gendered tensions underpinning North American advocacy efforts that seek to raise awareness and recognition of brain injuries among women participating in sport. This chapter draws upon accounts elicited through participant observation and interviews with advocates, clinicians, and researchers, which I collected as part of a larger project that examines how activism, regulatory discourses, and research coalesce in the framing of TBI as a health problem. The picture presented here is therefore not a comprehensive account of the scientific literature on or debates about sport-specific TBI among women. Rather, this chapter focuses on three domains of work carried out by advocates, clinicians, and researchers in order to elucidate the politics of sex/gender within each: (1) calls for sport-specific TBI policy and regulation; (2) explanations of sport-related TBI, and (3) scientific knowledge about TBI that informs—and is informed by—sport. After doing so, the conclusion offers a reflection on how different articulations of sex/gender operate constitutively in the shaping of concussion in women's sport *and* the female athlete as a body.

Distinguishing Women's Concussions in Sport as a Distinct Regulatory Issue

Many efforts to promote TBI awareness in women's sport contribute to and rely on rationalities and explanations that convey binary difference between men and women as a key dimension of TBI. They reflect a common tendency to frame sport-related injuries between men and women as distinct in which understandings—and subsequently, the treatment and rehabilitation—of women's injuries tend to emphasize physiological risk factors (Theberge 2015). In other domains, such as work settings, discussions about injuries are more often framed as the interplay between social and biological considerations (Theberge 2012). While both framings are potentially problematic in that they can posit social and biological factors as distinct instead of constitutive, the more integrated approach often employed to analyze workplace injuries is largely aspirational in relation to discussions of TBI in women's sports.

To distinguish how women's TBI is a unique problem, many advocates draw on popular narratives that make three main claims: (1) that female athletes suffer concussions at higher rates than their male counterparts in high school- and collegiate-level sport, (2) that they experience symptoms differently than men, and (3) that they require more time to recover from concussion than male athletes. Drawing attention to these particular concerns is a key strategy for raising awareness around the overlooked issue of TBI in women's sports, which is often overshadowed by the extensive coverage of the injury in relation to men's collision sports (e.g., Women's Sports Foundation 2015, 5, 10).[2]

Further review reveals that such claims, although common, often rely on the selective citation of research studies. One such analysis of data collected from 25 high schools suggests that even though male athletes accounted for the majority of documented concussions (due primarily to participation in football), girls playing soccer experienced concussions at double the rate of boys playing soccer (Lincoln et al. 2011). Cited studies of collegiate sport point to similar patterns, with women who play soccer and basketball seemingly suffering higher rates of concussions than their male counterparts and female softball players experiencing concussions at twice the rate of male baseball players (Hootman et al. 2007). Further, according to the authors of the same study, female ice hockey players, not male football players, had the highest rates of concussions in collegiate sport—a finding that has raised concerns from advocates and researchers alike.

On the one hand, these reports serve as grounds for drawing attention to the significance of TBI in women's sports as a health and welfare concern, because they seem to suggest higher rates of risk among women. On the other, as some researchers I interviewed for this study argued, stressing this particular finding can direct attention away from findings that show football players experience more concussions in competition *and* in practice. Both perspectives, however, do not raise questions about the nature of the evidence presented or the patterns of reporting—of which there is ample evidence that shows women participating in high school and university sport are more likely report TBI specifically and their injuries more generally (Miyashita et al. 2016; Kroshus et al. 2017; Mollayeva et al. 2018). Instead, the uncritical tendency to compare TBI rates in women's sports with men's sports reiterates an assumption of seemingly inherent binary differences in order to raise awareness of women's TBI.

Advocates I have spoken with tend to shy away from emphasizing the need to critically scrutinize patterns based on differential reporting, as the high rates of TBI among women are often the primary claim upon which they base calls for resources that can be used for awareness, education, and regulation. Expert recommendations and statements based on reviews of evidence, such as those put forth by the American Medical Society for Sports Medicine, reflect this tendency: Despite acknowledging the need for further research "to understand if sex is a risk factor for concussion and what mechanisms may account for it or if sex is merely a predictor of symptom reporting" (Harmon et al. 2013, 18), the Society's position statement dedicates comparatively more space to identifying biological differences related to sex as possible explanations for reported concussion rates. In particular, it cites disparities in head-neck size and strength, the role of sex hormones, and blood flow in and to the brain as possible explanatory factors that require further investigation (18). The statement, which frames its recommendations as expert advice, could thus be read in a way that reinscribes tacit beliefs about women's physical characteristics as core explanations for TBI in women—even though gendered variations in reporting are well known and there are noted shortcomings in existing epidemiological studies that do not adequately capture participants in women's sport (Resch et al. 2017).

These dynamics evince some of the tensions associated with so-called "evidence-based" approaches to sport governance (see Palmer 2013; Henne and Pape 2018). According to Catherine Palmer (2013), calls to use evidence as a guide for policy interventions in sport tend to frame evidence as if it is apolitical or value-free, even though policymakers often construct what counts as credible evidence through decision-making processes. In other words, what and how evidence becomes valued in policy spheres relies on subjective evaluations. In relation to the distinct challenges of assessing injury and bodily harm, criminologists Dawn Moore and Rashmee Singh's work on domestic violence cases offers important insights. It illustrates how modes of evaluating and corroborating evidence, even that which appears to be neutral (such as the visual documentation of a visible injury), are themselves interpretative practices informed by emotions and tacit beliefs (Moore and Singh 2018, 128–129). These processes often undermine victimized women's agency, as images generated and interpreted by more empowered actors, such as law enforcement officials, are often understood as more credible, even when a victim of intimate partner violence (who experienced the violence firsthand) offers alternative explanations (127). While TBI among athletes is a form of blunt force trauma that often occurs in very different settings, there are nonetheless parallels with Moore and Singh's observations: The interpretation of information in both contexts draws upon common scripts, which reflect "a related knowledge structure that enables us to make sense of things," and schemata, or organizing frameworks and "familiar stor[ies]," which aid in making causal inferences (Sherwin 1994, 50). Scientific insights and ideologies come together to have explanatory purchase when making sense of evidence.

Consider, for example, a recent comprehensive review of the literature on sport concussions among women (Resch et al. 2017). Despite pointing to inconsistencies and conflicting results from collected data, it supports conclusions that female athletes have an increased risk for concussion and that they report more severe symptoms than male athletes. Although the review acknowledges that the reasons for these differences remain inconclusive, it, like many other statements by advocates and researchers, does not shy away from offering speculative reasoning that evokes biological difference in an explanatory sense. As mentioned, the claim that girls and women tend to have less neck strength than boys and men, which makes their heads more prone to impact and trauma, is common (e.g., Collins et al. 2014). Others point to findings that hormonal changes linked to one's menstrual cycle phase can affect both the intensity and duration of TBI symptoms (Wunderle et al. 2014). In focusing on these concerns, efforts to raise awareness in the interests of women's health present risks to the brain as linked to inherent and universally shared attributes, presenting them as if they are rooted in presumptions of women's physical, and presumably weaker, difference.

These beliefs carry over into advocacy efforts that call for more scientific studies on women who have experienced concussions and preventive measures. Lobbying for greater focus on female athletes' experiences of TBI, however, can foreclose the interrogation of other gendered considerations that emerge in and beyond sport. For instance, because of the failure to reflect on how the quality of reporting around concussion symptoms implicates understandings of TBI, there is limited engagement with questions regarding athletes' perceptions of risk, pain, and injury, all of which have documented gendered *and* racialized contours according to U.S. studies (Nixon 1996).

These socio-cultural dimensions inform data collection, outcomes, and regulatory practices related to TBI. As the implementation of concussion protocols varies across sports, self-reporting is still a significant source of data on sports-related TBI. It is therefore reasonable to ascertain that men are more likely to under-report and that this pattern is linked to a cult of masculinity engendered through sport (Mollayeva et al. 2018). As such, the norms of men's sport actually contribute to the perception that women athletes are more prone to TBI than men, which advocates and researchers, in turn, interpret through a gendered lens that attributes these differences to women's bodies.

Furthermore, these explanations negate existing research that shows how athletes' social networks, interpersonal relationships, and other sport-specific conditions foster "cultures of risk" that encourage participants to play through injury (Nixon 1992). In fact, findings suggest that even the coaches who express care and concern for athletes' health convey expectations that encourage such risk-taking (Nixon 1994). These socio-cultural insights may offer explanations not yet explored by many advocates or researchers in the context of TBI and report. If we take sport cultures seriously, we should ask whether and how women's sports environments might be more conducive to reporting, which is not necessarily linked to gender; it could be linked to other pressures, such as perceived competitive or financial stakes. Also, related explanations may not be limited to athletes or their decision-making; they may instead involve spaces less beholden to commercialized masculine norms such as women's sport with coaches and support staff, thus potentially being more attentive to injuries and symptoms or taking additional caution around questions about athletes' well-being. In sum, the focus on women reporting more than men misses an opportunity to engage questions about other norms and practices that contribute to concussion, data collection, and reporting.

Explaining Concussion in Women's Sport

As part of the effort to raise awareness of TBI among women, many advocates see their work as explaining how and why their experiences are different from their male counterparts. Katherine Snedaker, founder of PINK Concussions, which is dedicated to raising awareness of and educating people about female brain injury, explains she created the organization "to improve the research, medical care, and community support for females with brain injury including concussion. . . . I believe females with brain injuries ARE the invisible patients within 'the invisible injury'."[3] In keeping with this focus, the organization's website draws attention to how "female and male brains differ in more than 100 ways in structure, activity, chemistry, and blood flow, and so it is logical that damage to the brain would also manifest differently in women and men."[4] Accordingly, the website text reflects some researchers' claim that there are "male and female brains," an assertion that has been challenged by more recent theories around brain plasticity, socialization, and observations that a brain "changes throughout life" (Pitts-Taylor 2016, 31). PINK Concussions is not alone in using this sex-based language to make claims about the specific needs of female bodies. Many explanations of TBI in women rely on rationales rooted in sex difference, which tend "to generate uniform, generalized accounts of male and female brains, traits, and behaviors, thereby obliterating the variations within each category, as well as those variations that call the two bifurcated categories into question" (Pitts-Taylor 2016, 119). These dominant explanations often fail to include qualifiers or express concerns about how some women (and gender identities) may have distinct vulnerabilities.

Instead of interrogating many of these nuanced distinctions, advocates and researchers tend to evoke the "female athlete" as a category of person which often emerges as one who is particularly vulnerable to TBI as a result of particular biological susceptibilities. For example, when a group of U.S. experts convened in late 2017 to identify and discuss important areas for future research, their discussion of sport-related recommendations reflected an appreciation of potentially relevant socio-cultural issues, but offered no details regarding how to connect them with biomedical findings informed by sex difference.[5] In fact, the workshop, although multidisciplinary in scope, disproportionately featured presentations encouraging more detailed analyses of internal brain processes and injury responses among female subjects, suggesting a narrower set of research priorities (the implications of which I discuss in the next section of this chapter). When those experts did acknowledge the need for more research on sport-specific concerns, they presented the following topics as priorities: the action of hormones in female concussed subjects, greater focus on needs-specific rehabilitation, and the need to expand studies to include sports and age groups beyond National Collegiate Athletic Association (NCAA) sports. They did not, however, speculate how these research priorities would complement each other in practice or how to study the dynamic social systems that contribute to TBI among women in sport.

Accordingly, calls for research can come with tradeoffs: they often evoke the need for more biomedical research and lose sight of wider contextual concerns. In doing so, they can over-emphasize such risks as specific to female anatomy. In short, they negate what sociologist Nancy Theberge (2012) describes as the more "complex interrelationship between biological and social sources of injuries and health hazards generally" (184). Explanations of injury that privilege physiological distinctions between men and women, she argues, tend to overlook sport-specific patterns or other social and material formations of difference. As a result, interventions may be targeted, but they tend to be limited. Consider, for instance, concerns around the prevalence of anterior cruciate ligament (ACL) injuries in female athletes—an issue that has garnered significant attention even though most ACL tears result from car accidents and are also common in men's tackle football. Years of gender-specific research and efforts to encourage biomechanical corrections to women's bodies have not significantly curtailed injury rates. While TBI is a distinctly different kind of injury compared to ACL tears and poses different challenges for those who experience it, attempts to understand both injuries discursively evoke an imagined universal female subject and her presumed differences and needs. Responses to both cases emphasize how these injuries are unique to women because of their physiology, even as proponents of women's sport have long refuted beliefs that female bodies are inherently weaker than—or dysfunctional compared to—male bodies. As Theberge (2012, 187) observes, presenting what are more complicated gender concerns as simply "biological risk factors" can raise "the specter of a revival of notions of female frailty and unsuitability for vigorous physical activity," despite greater participation in and acceptance of women's sport.

It would be a misnomer to suggest all advocacy around TBI in women's sports essentializes women by prioritizing sex difference. There are active efforts to counter tacit beliefs about fragility of female bodies and brains. The University of Minnesota Tucker Center for Research on Women and Girls in Sport, working with Twin Cities Public Television, has produced a documentary on concussions in women's sport. It attempts to highlight how gendered dimensions of women's sport participation may shape experiences of concussion, featuring expert commentaries that balance a range of considerations: competitive and sport-specific norms that can affect athletes' health and safety;

age-related, cognitive, and physiological, differences that can influence experiences of concussion; as well as wider regulatory and treatment challenges for administrators, coaches, referees, and support staff to consider critically. Some documentary commentators also address how media coverage often renders female bodies as more vulnerable to injury, which can serve as problematic grounds for rethinking the nature and extent of their participation in sport. In contrast, they state, coverage of men's concussion never sparks comparable reconsiderations of their bodily capacity, even though its public visibility is greater. In fact, the embrace of violence in men's collision sports arguably reinforces beliefs that men are naturally stronger and more resilient than female athletes. The emphasis on the higher rates of TBI in women's collision sports, such as hockey, seemingly reifies this point, especially when the citation of these rates fails to account for women's higher rates of reporting. In response to these concerns, the documentary concludes by advocating for more multidisciplinary inquiry into how concussion symptoms and health outcomes can vary greatly by individual, irrespective of gender, and to examine how societal and sport-specific conditions may contribute to making participants in women's sports more vulnerable to TBI.

The documentary's recommendations align with a vocal minority of experts observed in my own research. For instance, in a TBI agenda-setting meeting, one researcher dedicated a presentation to explaining the importance of studying broader patterns of difference in sports-related concussion, stating explicitly that "we must use epidemiological data to drive prevention efforts so that we can keep athletes as safe as possible while they get the benefit of that physical activity while playing sports."[6] She framed prevention as a necessary priority: "I know if I prevent that direct blow—that direct transfer of force to the head—or the blow to the body . . . that causes the acceleration/deceleration of the rotational forces of the brain within the skull, [we] can prevent the concussion." Importantly, she contended, "Primary prevention efforts largely are just as effective in female athletes as they are male athletes, whether it's banning heading [the ball in soccer] or eliminating athlete-athlete contact or putting a helmet on both girls and boys lacrosse players." In other words, sports, by being rule-based, offer multiple opportunities for intervention. In fact, as the speaker elaborated, the same data showing the existence of differences between how men and women experience concussion symptoms also illustrates that those gaps are shrinking, which may suggest that post-concussion identification and treatment protocols have an impact. As such, her observations indicate that the rates of reporting—not the rates of concussion—are important gendered distinctions in terms of documenting TBI.

Despite these more promising signs, available population-level data only reveal certain kinds of differences, which are primarily framed in binary terms between male and female athletes. Such data do not provide information on the diverse subgroups that make up those larger comparative groups, an issue about which the same workshop participant expressed concern. The absence of more granular data prevents fine-grained analysis. Because of this shortcoming, she acknowledged, researchers actually knew little about the social contours of risk, even as they claimed to identify TBI risk factors among individuals. The lack of data, in turn, contributes to reifying the centrality of differences between women and men while minimizing—even arguably *invisibilizing*—other distinctions, such as socio-economic and racialized inequalities or resources linked to geographic location. Further, only one speaker at the aforementioned meeting of experts drew attention to these specific considerations and how they could enhance approaches to understanding concussion risk among athletes. It was therefore not surprising to learn that researchers lacked accessible data on concussions among transgender or intersex athletes, despite the growing numbers of openly transgender athletes participating in high school and collegiate sports in North America. Rendering these athletes invisible within discussions of TBI in sport reflects the historical preoccupation with protecting " 'fully' female athletes" under the guise that they are the weaker sex, which has led to the exclusion of athletes who do not fit within imagined feminine constructs (Henne 2014, 799). This history also shows us, as I have argued elsewhere (Henne 2014), there is no singular or clear biological marker that distinguishes women from men. Calls that focus on female TBI thus can perpetuate myths about gendered difference as they attempt to isolate female attributes associated with concussion risk.

The lack of data on TBI among diverse athletes similarly reflects and contributes to gendered understandings of sport, as it prevents accounting for bodies that do not fit binary ideal types or dismisses their diversity so as to render them into ideal types. As Pitts-Taylor (2016, 59) reminds us, bodies, "regularly run afoul of neat categorization"; an ideal body "has to be recognized as such; it is not a real, living, enacting, or perceiving body, but a construct." Rather than rely on ideals, she argues, "[s]ocial inequalities and power relations *should* be brought to bear on how we think about the brain, mind, and body, and neuroscientific accounts need to be cognizant of the different ways that power and inequality can affect lives" (124). Not only does the commitment to understanding female TBI seem to undermine those objectives, my research also suggests that even fields of study that are attentive to socio-cultural conditions, such as social epidemiology, still do not attend to how other social inequalities may help to explain observed differences in experiences of concussion. Instead, the preoccupation with differences between men and women remains the mainstay of gendered understandings of TBI, overlooking how other axes and assemblages of difference come to shape and mediate concussion among participants in sport, as well as the quality of their diagnosis and treatment.

Significant questions remain regarding how interlocking relationships between inequality and social difference inform experiences of TBI both within and beyond sport. Existing research on men's collision sports points to patterns in which race, for example, are directly relevant considerations. Analyses reveal that athletes from racialized backgrounds have often found themselves channeled into sport-specific positions that are considered non-leadership roles and often require greater levels of physical contact or more bodily risk-taking, which could contribute to higher rates of TBI (see Hokowhitu 2004; Moore 2015; Siler 2019). Additionally, research on health disparities illustrates that race and socio-economic inequality have a cumulative effect on mental and physical health outcomes in the United States. Race-related discrimination is therefore a particular concern because "its threat may be more systematic, insidious, and constant than other stressors" on health (Williams and Mohammed 2009, 31). In fact, public health research demonstrates that social forces manifest in racial minority bodies. This is especially the case within the stress paradigm where racialized minorities are thought to experience a distinct "*allostatic load*, or the cumulative wear and tear on the body's systems owing to repeated adaptation to stressors," including racism, which contributes to health deterioration earlier in life compared to whites (Geronimus et al. 2006, 826).

The limited TBI research attentive to race points to racial disparities in health outcomes following injury (Williams et al. 2009). Despite these observations of how racism uniquely contributes to and exacerbates health disparities, such concerns remain largely absent from the discourse of TBI in women's sport, because the focus on "female athletes" prioritizes sex/gender—and sex more so than gender—as the primary lens for distinguishing differences in TBI-related symptoms and experiences. This focus reveals a classic intersectional dilemma: As explained by Kimberlé Crenshaw (1991), focusing on one axis of social difference (in this case, sex/gender) tends to overlook and misrepresent the experiences of women of color who experience forms of marginalization that exceed the scope of sex/gender. In relation to health disparities, Joe Fagin and Zinobia Bennefield (2014) explicitly state that the ways black women have borne the brunt of systemic racism in U.S. health care often goes overlooked, even though it can be traced from historical forms of dehumanization to contemporary practices of mistreatment. These patterns can be observed in sport-related cases as well. For example, tennis star Serena Williams's documented struggle to receive treatment for dangerous complications following childbirth reveals that even elite Black female athletes can experience distinct health-related discrimination when seeking medical care.[7] Yet, intersectionality still receives little attention in TBI-related advocacy in sport. With these concerns in mind, the next section examines how the politics of sex difference play out in relation to scientific knowledge, attending to how they carry over into understandings of sport-specific TBI among women.

Relationships Between Scientific Knowledge of Female TBI and Sport

As expressed concerns around female athletes invite biologized explanations of the injury, they also convey a desire for more—and more nuanced—research that is attentive to how women's bodies and brains are distinct. In this case, preoccupations with the "female" dimension of TBI in women's sports come to fore, but knowledge about the "female athlete" comes from an amalgamation of clinical and preclinical scientific research, available evidence, and tacit knowledge about sex/gender. A meeting aimed at mapping out a research agenda setting for TBI in women revealed how the National Institutes of Health (NIH) policy on the inclusion of sex as a biological variable reaffirms this focus on male/female difference. As women make up approximately half of NIH-funded clinical research participants, the agency sought to ensure what it describes as the "adequate consideration of both sexes" by providing guidelines that specify the inclusion of "sex as a biological variable" in response to "the over-reliance on male animals and cells" in pre-clinical biomedical research (NIH Office of Research on Women's Health 2018).[8] The NIH policy, while heralded by some (e.g., Klein et al. 2015), attracted criticism for purporting sex-based likenesses across dissimilar species despite the absence of evidence to support that link, as it may "introduce conceptual and empirical errors into research" (Richardson et al. 2015).

Another potential tradeoff is how the NIH policy reinscribes biological difference as important and distinct, implying that sex can be isolated and distinguished from other gendered, material, or social considerations. These issues emerged most clearly when researchers and advocates met to assess the state of health-related research on TBI in women and to outline future research priorities. Many participants made sure to articulate their understandings of the distinctions between conceptions of sex and gender. To quote one participant considered an expert on sex differences:

> [G]ender is a purely human construct. . . . I have a lot of colleagues who like to argue with me about whether animals have gender. . . . But to this point, we pretty much are in agreement that animals, if they do have gender, they can't tell us. So, our quest to improve sex as a biological variable usage is to get the reviewers of journal articles to remind researchers that [if] you're [studying] animals you are studying sex.[9]

The statement was not unique in terms of charactering laboratory animals as lacking gender, reflecting broader norms around how such animals are often thought of technologies within biomedical systems of pursuing knowledge (Shew and Johnson 2018). In the context of the meetings, pre-clinical research emerged as the site for finding insights unique to biological sex—with animals serving an instrumental purpose for extracting such knowledge. Despite some statements about the interplay between sex and gender, participants' language about how they studied sex—and did not intend to study gender—rendered sex as the central lens for research priorities related to TBI in women, even though women live in social worlds in which sex/gender are inextricably linked. As such, their narratives articulated a binary between female and male and between sex and gender.

The move to draw distinctions between sex and gender has unforeseen implications, some of which are directly applicable for dominant understandings of TBI in women. Rarely did participants problematize the distinctions drawn or acknowledge their constitutive character—even as some experts expressed concerns that many phase three trials on TBI fail, as the findings observed in animal models do not translate to human studies. This prompted meeting participants' reflections on the challenges of preclinical research in this area, given that female mice may offer few insights into human sex difference due to their hormonal, reproductive, and sexual dissimilarities. However, the proposed solution was to embrace large animal models, such as pigs, as subjects. As explained by one participant, doing so would enable the examination of more complex pathophysiology, including more TBI-specific variables while also supporting the refinement of surgical procedures. As these examples illustrate, preclinical research received significant attention in terms of time dedicated to formal presentations about TBI-related studies, therefore a focus on sex over gender tended to dominate the meeting.

The privileging of sex over gender or other social categories of difference carried over into reflections on clinical, epidemiological, and rehabilitation studies. During discussions about clinical trials, participants acknowledged the under-representation of women versus men in TBI studies as another shortcoming that hindered the viability of translational research. Their observations conveyed a preoccupation with the inclusion of women, with relatively little attention paid to how other material conditions could—or should—be accounted for. Instead, many verbalized critiques oriented around the number and percentage of women in studies and the nature of observable differences as compared to men, rather than whether or not and how research designs could be modified to attend to intersectional considerations. Questions of social context reflected a similarly narrow scope, with an emphasis on individual behavior, which one expert framed as the "place where biological sex, cultural gender, self-expression, personal outward expressions of identity, sexual orientation—all these things are really mixed together."[10] Although an epidemiologist had raised questions about the role of other dimensions of social location, such as the issues of age, race/ethnicity, immigration or socioeconomic status, and sexual orientation, most participants concerned with social difference instead reiterated the importance of isolated "amalgamation of biological sex and gender identity and gender expression."[11] Moreover, they usually called for experimental or quasi-experimental designs that aim to isolate causal relationships. Overall, the influence of the NIH policy is notable in that binary sex/gender—and more sex than gender—became a central focus. This maneuver is insidious, although likely unintended, given that the justification for the policy on the inclusion of sex as a biological variable is the pursuit of more equitable health outcomes for women.

The preoccupation with sex difference carried over into discussions of women with TBI, including athletes. Again, the emphasis on biological considerations arose as central across discussions of human studies, especially around sex hormones and the menstrual cycle in women. Specifically, scientists would point to research which indicates that women with raised levels of progesterone at the time of injury often have better outcomes than women who have high levels of estrogen when injured. Progesterone is also a possible treatment for women who are struggling with TBI symptoms, something one advocate described as saving her from "unbearable pain where I've felt my head separate from my body every single month. . . . [W]ithin a few weeks of having a natural progesterone cream that I rubbed into my head every day, twice a day, it was the first time I actually got rid of my migraines." Many researchers described these findings as having breakthrough implications, seemingly justifying the power and potential of research attentive to sex difference. This focus lends to TBI-related interventions that primarily target internal bodily dynamics, rather than social forces or sport-specific dynamics.

Science does not simply inform understandings of TBI in women in ways that carry over into sport; sport also informs the science of TBI in women. During the same agenda-setting meeting, many participants acknowledged that scientific knowledge about TBI relies heavily on studies of sport participants and the resources being channeled into sport-specific research, particularly from private corporate entities like the National Football League (NFL). The military, too, has provided significant support for TBI research, developing partnerships with sports organizations, such as the NCAA-Department of Defense (DoD) CARE consortium, in order to conduct larger, comparative studies. The CARE consortium, for example, is currently undertaking the most comprehensive and longitudinal study of concussion in athletes and military cadets carried out to date. In contrast, researchers working on issues of TBI in women as a result of domestic violence expressed frustration that they had significantly less funding. Although recognizing this particular gap, few scientists posed questions about the potential shortcomings of an evidence base that relies primarily on findings that privilege younger and more active participants who were likely to be in good or better than average health prior to experiencing one or more TBIs. And, sex again emerged as a privileged mode through which to make sense of TBI among women, even though athletes and military personnel are not representative of other groups of women who experience concussion.

Discussion and Conclusion

Overall, the aforementioned agenda-setting activities for research on TBI in women indicate two key areas for consideration. First, they showcase how forms of biological reductionism centered around female bodies become entrenched almost paradoxically through the recognition of sex/gender. In doing so, the focus on sex difference forecloses greater consideration of what public health scholars frame as "social determinants of health"—a term that draws attention to how growing inequalities yield disproportionate health outcomes for marginalized populations (see Marmot et al. 2008). Second, they perpetuate beliefs about female athletes as not only being fundamentally different than male athletes, but also weaker or deficient by comparison—myths that also disregard the diversity of athlete bodies and sport cultures. Taken together, both issues reveal that studies of TBI run the risk of privileging "[b]iological narratives about human (and nonhuman animal) experience," which, as Pitts-Taylor (2016, 119) cautions, can "deny the complexity, specificity, and multiplicity of lives."

The framing of female bodies as central to understanding TBI in women's sport reflects a set of politics that Sally Engle Merry and Susan Coutin (2014, 12) explain as being inextricably linked to how " 'problems' are identified and made known in the first place." Developing knowledge about and responding to social problems often means considerations that are "too hard to categorize and classify may not be discerned at all," and "complex social ties" are often erased in an appeal for measurable and seemingly objective forms of evidence (Merry and Coutin 2014, 12). Thus, while it is understandable and important not to dismiss TBI among women within the wider discussion of sports' concussion crises, it is also essential to consider the tradeoffs that accompany its framing as a social problem. For example, the establishment of new initiatives that purport to close gaps in knowledge about TBI often fail to consider how multiple gaps, not simply one between men and women, co-exist. The promotion of the newly established Female Brain Bank, a partnership between the National Posttraumatic Stress Disorder (PTSD) Brain Bank (funded by the U.S. Department of Veterans Affairs) and PINK Concussions offers a case in point. Similar to the VA-BU-CLF Brain Bank, which is the largest tissue repository in the world dedicated to the study of TBI and chronic traumatic encephalopathy (CTE), it accepts posthumous brain donations with a particular aim of redressing the lack of female brains available for research. While the Female Brain Bank has been praised for ensuring that studies account for sex differences evinced through the study of brains from women who have suffered TBI, it has the potential to offer other kinds of insights, as Female Brain Bank has actively encouraged a diverse sample of women donors. Whether or not and how researchers capture that diversity, however, is not yet known.

What is known is that the director of the NIH Office of Research on Women's Health, Dr. Janine Clayton, has strongly advocated for the "Sex as a Biological Variable" policy, framing it as a necessary reform to ensure better health outcomes for women. This stance positions sex difference in a way that benefits not only from scientific authority and governmental backing, but also from the credibility often afforded to those institutions. In contrast, this chapter marks an initial step in thinking through the selective and strategic (in)visibility of gender that emerges when sex difference becomes the primary lens through which to understand women's injuries and health. As such, this analysis points to at least one critical implication of these well-intended efforts: that they can actually work in the service of hegemonically reifying the divide between women and men as seemingly based on natural—as opposed to naturalized—sex difference (see Henne 2014).

This case reveals how the preoccupation with TBI in female athletes highlights articulations of sex/gender that inform the mutual shaping of concussion in women's sport *and* the female athlete as a body. To borrow from Mol (2003), female TBI and the female athlete come into being together through a collaboration of sex/gender, advocacy, science, and sport, which work in concert through attempts to address the social problem of TBI in women's sport. The assertion of "female TBI" as a thing backed by science emerges as a gendered creation that is constituted in part from imagined characteristics that become attributed to sex. Accordingly, efforts to understand concussion among female athletes do more than evoke an ideal body in their framings of TBI; the knowledge base materializes in a way that suggests these ideal female athlete bodies are natural phenomena, even though Pitts-Taylor (2016) reminds us they are socially created.

Notes

1. Historically, sex has been relegated to the biological features, including sex organs and chromosomes, while gender suggests cultural constructions that include feminine and masculine attributes. The distinctions between sex and gender, however, are contested. Dussauge and Kaiser (2012, 212) acknowledge that "feminist neuroscientists are still working to define an appropriate vocabulary for what is not inseparable but interlaced, not fixed but alterable." Thus, in many places in this chapter, I use "sex/gender" to flag these complicated dynamics.
2. See also, for example: "Female Brain Injury." *PINK Concussions.* www. pinkconcussions.com/new-page-1
3. "Katherine Price Snedaker, LCSW, Executive Director." *PINK Concussions.* www.pinkconcussions.com/about
4. "Female Brain Injury." *PINK Concussions.* www.pinkconcussions.com/ new-page-1
5. Field notes, December 19, 2017. Recognizing this challenge, Mollayeva and colleagues (2018, 2) identify the "explicit and consistent consideration of the interrelated constructs of sex and gender in TBI research" as an important avenue for future research.
6. Field notes, December 18, 2017.
7. Black women in the United States are three to four times more likely than their white counterparts to die from pregnancy-related complications, regardless of socioeconomic status, a concern that many commentators attribute to both overt and discursive forms of discrimination as well as racialized health stressors (Gay 2018).
8. This approach is specific to the United States. For example, the Canadian Institutes of Health Research (CIHR) outline expectations "that all research applicants will integrate gender and sex into their research designs when appropriate" in order "to make health research more just, more rigorous, and more useful" (CIHR 2017).
9. Field notes, December 18, 2017.
10. Ibid., December 19, 2017.
11. Ibid.

References

Canadian Institutes of Health Research. 2017. *Sex, Gender and Health Research Guide: A Tool for CIHR Applicants.* www.cihr-irsc.gc.ca/e/32019.html

Centers for Disease Control and Prevention. 2019. *Surveillance Report of Traumatic Brain Injury-related Emergency Department Visits, Hospitalizations, and Deaths—United States, 2014.* Atlanta, Georgia: U.S. Department of Health and Human Services.

Collins, Christy L., Erica N. Fletcher, Sarah K. Fields, Lisa Kluchurosky, Mary Kay Rohrkemper, R. Dawn Comstock, and Robert C. Cantu. 2014. "Neck Strength: A Protective Factor Reducing Risk for Concussion in High School Sports." *The Journal of Primary Prevention* 35 (5): 309–319.

Crenshaw, Kimberlé W. 1991. "Mapping the Margins: Intersectionality, Identity Politics, and Violence Against Women of Color." *Stanford Law Review* 43 (6): 1241–1299.

Dussauge, Isabelle, and Anelis Kaiser. 2012. "Neuroscience and Sex/Gender." *Neuroethics* 5 (1): 211–215.

Fagin, Joe, and Zinobia Bennefield. 2014. "Systemic Racism and U.S. Health Care." *Social Science & Medicine* 103 (1): 7–14.

Fausto-Sterling, Anne. 2005. "The Bare Bones of Sex: Part 1—Sex and Gender." *Signs: Journal of Women and Culture in Society* 30 (2): 1491–1527.

Gary, Kelli W., Juan Carlos Arango-Lasprilla, and Lilian Flores Stevens. 2009. "Do Racial/Ethnic Differences Exist in Post-Injury Outcomes After TBI? A Comprehensive Review of the Literature." *Brain Injury* 23 (10): 775–789.

Gay, Elizabeth Dawes. 2018. "Serena Williams Could Insist that Doctors Listen to Her. Most Black Women Can't." *The Nation*, January 18. www.thenation.com/article/serena-williams-could-insist-that-doctors-listen-to-her-most-black-women-cant/

Geronimus, Arline T., Margaret Hicken, Danya Keene, and John Bound. 2006. "'Weathering' and Age Patterns of Allostatic Load Scores Among Blacks and Whites in the United States." *American Journal of Public Health* 96 (5): 826–833.

Hargreaves, Jennifer. 1994. *Sporting Females: Critical Issues in the History and Sociology of Women's Sport*. London: Routledge.

Harmon, Kimberly G., Jonathan A. Drezner, Matthew Gammons, Kevin M. Guskiewicz, Mark Halstead, Stanley A. Herring, Jeffrey S. Kutcher, Andrea Pana, Margot Putukian, and William O. Roberts. 2013. "American Medical Society for Sports Medicine Position Statement: Concussion in Sport." *British Journal of Sports Medicine* 47: 15–26.

Henne, Kathryn. 2014. "The 'Science' of Fair Play in Sport: Gender and the Politics of Testing." *Signs* 39 (3): 767–812.

Henne, Kathryn, and Madeleine Pape. 2018. "Dilemmas of Gender and Global Sports Governance: An Invitation to Southern Theory." *Sociology of Sport Journal* 35 (3): 216–225.

Hokowhitu, Brendan. 2004. "Tackling Māori Masculinity: A Colonial Genealogy of Savagery and Sport." *The Contemporary Pacific* 16 (2): 259–284.

Hootman, Jennifer M., Randall Dick, and Julie Agel. 2007. "Epidemiology of Collegiate Injuries for 15 Sports: Summary and Recommendations for Injury Prevention Initiatives." *Journal of Athletic Training* 42 (2): 311–319.

Jordan-Young, Rebecca. 2011. *Brain Storm: The Flaws in the Science of Sex Differences*. Cambridge, MA: Harvard University Press.

Klein, Sabra L., Londa Schiebinger, Marcia L. Stefanick, Larry Cahill, Jayne Danska, Geert J. de Vries, Melina R. Kibbe, Margaret M. McCarthy, Jeffrey S. Mogil, Teresa K. Woodruff, et al. 2015. "Sex Inclusion in Basic Research Drives Discovery." *Proceedings of the National Academy of Sciences of the United States of America* 112 (17): 5257–5258.

Kroshus, Emily, Christine M. Baugh, Cynthia J. Stein, S. Bryn Austin, and Jerel P. Calzo. 2017. "Concussion Reporting, Sex, and Conformity to Traditional Gender Norms in Young Adults." *Journal of Adolescence* 54: 110–119.

Lamke, Sherece. 2011. *Concussion and Female Athletes: The Untold Story.* http://video.tpt.org/video/2260739330/

Lincoln, Andrew E., Shane V. Caswell, Jon L. Almquist, Reginald E. Dunn, Joseph B. Norris, and Richard Y. Hinton. 2011. "Trends in Concussion Incidence in High School Sports: A Prospective 11-year Study." *The American Journal of Sports Medicine* 39 (5): 958–963.

Marmot, Michael., Sharon Friel, Ruth Bell, R., Tanya A.J. Houweling, and Sebastian Taylor. 2008. "Closing the Gap in a Generation: Health Equity Through Action on the Social Determinants of Health." *The Lancet* 372 (9650): 1661–1669.

Merry, Sally Engle, and Susan Bibler Coutin. 2014. "Technologies of Truth in the Anthropology of Conflict." *American Ethnologist* 41 (1): 1–16.

Miyashita, Theresa L., Eleni Diakogeorgiou, and Christina VanderVegt. 2016. "Gender Differences in Concussion Reporting Among High School Athletes." *Sports Health* 8: 359–363.

Mol, Annemarie. 2003. *The Body Multiple: Ontology in Medical Practice.* Durham, NC: Duke University Press.

Mollayeva, Tatyana, Shirin Mollayeva, and Angela Colantonio. 2018. "Traumatic Brain Injury: Sex, Gender, and Intersecting Vulnerabilities." *Nature Reviews* 14: 711–722.

Moore, Antonio. 2015. "Football's War on the Minds of Black Men." *Vice Sports,* December 24. https://sports.vice.com/en_us/article/eze4gj/footballs-war-on-the-minds-of-black-men

Moore, Dawn, and Rashmee Singh. 2018. "Seeing Crime, Feeling Crime: Visual Evidence, Emotions, and the Prosecution of Domestic violence." *Theoretical Criminology* 22 (1): 116–132.

National Institutes of Health Office of Research on Women's Health. 2018. *NIH Policy on Sex as a Biological Variable.* https://orwh.od.nih.gov/research/sex-gender/nih-policy/

Nixon, Howard L. 1992. "A Social Network Analysis of Influences on Athletes to Play with Pain and Injuries." *Journal of Sport & Social Issues* 16 (2): 127–135.

Nixon, Howard L. 1994. "Coaches' Views of Risk, Pain, and Injury in Sport, with Special Reference to Gender Differences." *Sociology of Sport Journal* 11 (1): 79–87.

Nixon, Howard L. 1996. "Explaining Pain and Injury Attitudes and Experiences in Sport in Terms of Gender, Race, and Sport Status." *Journal of Sport & Social Issues* 20 (2): 33–44.

Palmer, Catherine. 2013. *Global Sports Policy.* London: Sage.

Pitts-Taylor, Victoria. 2016. *The Brain's Body: Neuroscience and Corporeal Politics.* Durham, NC: Duke University Press.

Puar, Jasbir K. 2012. "'I Would Rather be a Cyborg than a Goddess': Becoming-Intersectional in Assemblage Theory." *Philosophia* 2 (1): 49–66.

Resch, Jacob E., Amanda Rach, Samuel Walton, and Donna K. Broshek. 2017. "Sport Concussion and the Female Athlete." *Clinics in Sport Medicine* 36 (4): 717–739.

Richardson, Sarah S., Meredith Reiches, Heather Shattuck-Heidorn, Michelle L. LaBonte, and Theresa Consoli. 2015. "Focus on Preclinical Sex Differences Will Not Address Women's and Men's Health Disparities." *Proceedings of the National Academy of Sciences of the United States of America* 112 (44): 13419–13420.

Roy, Deboleena. 2016. "Neuroscience and Feminist Theory: A New Directions Essay." *Signs* 41 (3): 531–552.

Sharpe, David J., and Peter O. Jenkins. 2015. "Concussion is Confusing Us All." *Practical Neurology* 15 (3): 172–186.

Sherwin, Richard K. 1994. "Law Frames: Historical Truth and Narrative Necessity in a Criminal Case." *Stanford Law Review* 47 (1): 39–84.

Shew, Ashley, and Keith Johnson. 2018. "Companion Animals as Technologies in Biomedical Research." *Perspectives on Science* 26 (3): 400–417.

Siler, Kyle. 2019. "Pipelines on the Gridiron: Player Backgrounds, Opportunity Structures and Racial Stratification in American College Football." *Sociology of Sport Journal* 36 (1): 57–76.

Subramaniam, Banu. 2009. "Moored Metamorphoses: A Retrospective Essay on Feminist Science Studies." *Signs* 34 (4): 951–980.

Tagge, Chad A., Andrew M. Fisher, Olga V. Minaeva, Amanda Gaudreau-Balderrama, Juliet A. Moncaster, Xiao-Lei Zhang, Mark W. Wojnarowicz, et al. 2018. "Concussion, Microvascular Injury, and Early Tauopathy in Young Athletes After Impact Head Injury and an Impact Concussion Mouse Model." *Brain* 141: 422–458.

Theberge, Nancy. 2012. "Studying Gender and Injuries: A Comparative Analysis of the Literature on Women's Injuries in Sport and Work." *Ergonomics* 55 (2): 183–193.

Theberge, Nancy. 2015. "Social Sources of Research Interest in Women's Sport Related Injuries: A Case Study of ACL Injuries." *Sociology of Sport Journal* 32 (3): 229–247.

Trujillo, Nick. 1995. "Machines, Missiles, and Men: Images of the Male Body on ABC's Monday Night Football." *Sociology of Sport Journal* 12 (4): 403–423.

Ventresca, Matt. 2019. "The Curious Case of CTE: Mediating Materialities of Traumatic Brain Injury." *Communication & Sport* 7 (2): 135–156.

Vertinsky, Patricia. 1987. "Exercise, Physical Capability, and the Eternally Wounded Woman in Late Nineteenth Century North America." *Journal of Sport History* 14 (1): 7–27.

Williams, David R., and Selina A. Mohammed. 2009. "Discrimination and Racial Disparities in Health: Evidence and Needed Research." *Journal of Behavioral Medicine* 32 (1): 20–47.

Women's Sports Foundation. 2015. *Her Life Depends on It III: Sport, Physical Activity, and the Health and Well-Being of American Girls and Women*. www.womenssportsfoundation.org/research/article-and-report/recent-research/her-life-depends-on-it-iii/

Wunderle, Kathryn, Kathleen Hoeger, Erin Wasserman, and Jeffrey Bazarian. 2014. "Menstrual Phase as Predictor of Outcome After Mild Traumatic Brain Injury in Women." *The Journal of Head Trauma Rehabilitation* 29 (5): E1–E8.

10 Beyond the Biopsychosocial

A Case for Critical Qualitative Concussion Research

Matt Ventresca

Contemporary approaches to concussion diagnosis and treatment commonly advocate for care administered by multidisciplinary teams of medical professionals. These teams tend to include neuropsychologists, neurologists, physiotherapists, psychiatrists, exercise scientists, sports medicine physicians, and athletic therapists (Panczykowski and Pardini 2014). The broad disciplinary scope of concussion management programs stems not only from the complex multifaceted nature of the injury, but also from the limits of imaging techniques or physiological tests to definitively detect neuropathological changes characteristic of concussion. Given their focus on relationships between brain and behaviour, neuropsychologists have been especially central to the design and application of standardized tests for *indirectly* measuring the course and severity of concussive injuries. These tests are unique in how they are designed to assess psychological variables (cognition, emotions, etc.) in addition to physical symptoms such as headache, balance, or dizziness. The subdiscipline of sports neuropsychology has emerged around the need to study sport-specific mechanisms of concussive injuries and ways ultra-competitive sport contexts influence psychological responses to diagnosis or recovery (Webbe 2010; Echemendia and Julian 2001).

The principles for multidimensional treatment of concussion are often drawn from the *biopsychosocial model* of health and illness (Wäljas et al. 2015; McCrea et al. 2015; Silverberg et al. 2015). The model was popularized by psychiatrist George L. Engel, who in 1977 published an article in *Science* highlighting how the dominance of biomedical ways of knowing in psychology devalued the psychosocial aspects of illness and disease. Engel opposed how common approaches within biomedicine often reduce complex psychological processes to matters of biological dysfunction or neurochemical imbalances. He argued that a more comprehensive psychiatric assessment "must take into account the patient, the social context in which he [sic] lives, and the complementary system devised by society to deal with disruptive effects of illness" (132). The popularity of the biopsychosocial model across health fields has indeed created space for institutional definitions of health and illness to include mental and social factors alongside physiological variables.

Since concussion cannot be conclusively detected through "objective" biomedical tests or neuroimaging, the biopsychosocial model enables assessment of multiple variables that may indicate that a brain injury has occurred. These variables include "psychosocial" elements such as experiences of stress, depression, or anxiety, quality of social support, and individual expectations or motivations for recovery (McCrea et al. 2015). The biopsychosocial model of concussion also takes pre-injury factors into consideration, such as genetics, previous brain injuries, mental health history, and individual personality traits (Iverson 2012; Wäljas et al. 2015). The model, then, importantly challenges forms of neuroreductionism (Vidal and Ortega 2011) that advance limited conceptions of human behaviors as simply matters of brain function.

Yet the model has been shown to have distinct theoretical and methodological limitations. Many of these limitations emanate from philosophical assumptions about the nature of human life, especially in regard to the ways in which injury or illness disrupts the operations of an otherwise well-functioning system (Crossley 2008; Lima et al. 2014; Stam 2000; Bendelow 2009). Critical health scholars argue that the model works to erroneously compartmentalize lived experiences of health and illness into isolated variables which can presumably be individually quantified and measured (Stam 2000; Crossley 2008). These larger critiques coincide with specific arguments challenging the dominance of quantitative methodologies in the realm of concussion evaluation and how an over-reliance on scientific techniques works to discredit lay knowledge of injury experiences (Caron et al. 2013; Malcolm 2017; Ventresca, 2020). Such concerns have facilitated a steady growth of qualitative research into the complexity of athletes' lived experiences of concussion (Bridel et al. this volume; Liston et al. 2016; Todd et al. 2018; Caron et al. 2013; Moreau et al. 2014).

The purpose of this chapter is to critically examine the prominence of the biopsychosocial model in conceptions of sports concussion and traumatic brain injury (TBI). My analysis draws attention to limitations of the biopsychosocial model as a theoretical and methodological framework, while highlighting important roles for critical qualitative research in moving toward more complex conceptions of concussion. I investigate these directions through four related questions: *1) Why quantification (and why not)? 2) Why qualitative research? 3) Why experience? and 4) Is functionalism a fatal flaw?* Through these questions I interrogate the onto-epistemological foundations of the biopsychosocial model, making visible its limitations and challenging its primacy as a way of conceptualizing and managing concussion.

I argue that, despite its promise as an integrated approach to concussion, in practice the biopsychosocial model commonly reinforces the fallacy that scientific experiments and statistical techniques can neatly divide human experience into separate components. I demonstrate that, while the model's consideration of psychosocial variables seemingly *enables a better understanding of embodied concussion experiences, it too often produces narrow conceptions of these experiences as sums of their component parts.* I highlight how critical qualitative research provides methods for documenting and contextualizing athlete experiences of concussion that, importantly, situate these experiences within broader socio-historical processes. Yet I also explain that critical qualitative analysis reveals how seemingly different aspects of concussion are co-constructed and emerge together through embodied experiences of injury. I conclude the chapter by pointing toward alternative, interdisciplinary ways of knowing that resist the compartmentalization of human experience.

Why Quantification (and Why Not)?

The biopsychosocial model is primarily organized according to the logics of *functionalism*, which construct human life as constituted by complex interdependent systems. Under functionalist paradigms, bodies, ecosystems, and societies are made up of components that ideally work together to maintain effective operation of broader systems such as human bodies; that is, each component has an established function within the body and malfunctioning components will disrupt the system's—or body's—cohesiveness (Stam 2000; Crossley 2008; Bendelow 2009). Functionalism posits that understanding biological and social phenomena requires analyzing relationships between component parts that are apparently predictable and thus can be measured empirically. This assumption encourages the representation of biological processes and social behavior as quantifiable units of analysis that can be directly "inputted" into pre-existing conceptual models. Functionalism allows for the construction of health and illness as constituted by sets of pre-determined *variables* that can be evaluated and compared through statistical analysis (Crossley 2008; Stam 2000). Statistical calculations can then identify specific malfunctioning or under-performing components of the body and support strategic interventions to correct these problems. While functionalism is historically foundational to the scientific study of biological systems, critics of the paradigm have voiced concerns about its predominance within social science disciplines such as psychology and sociology (Crossley 2008; Stam 2000; Smith 1975).

Reflecting the paradigm's widespread influence within the life sciences, a functionalist conception of concussion was formalized through the development of the Sport as Laboratory Assessment Model (SLAM) at the University of Virginia in the 1980s. SLAM was designed to capitalize on how competitive sports contexts offer opportunities to closely monitor a clinical population both *before and after* injury (Barth et al. 2010). The logic of SLAM is that, unlike the general population, athletes are easily identifiable as individuals with significant risk of brain injury. It is therefore feasible to conduct pre-injury testing of physiological, cognitive, and psychological indicators with athletes to establish quantified "baseline" measures that can be compared to post-injury data. The differences in measurements could then be used to determine types of functioning impacted by brain injury and the scope and severity of these impairments. As its name implies, the proposed benefits of SLAM stem from the simulation of laboratory conditions; individual athletes serve as their own control when individual baseline measurements are compared to post-injury scores. In other words, the same athlete will simultaneously act as a member of the "healthy" and injured populations, offering a unique opportunity for controlled side-by-side comparisons of change over time. Given its systematic approach to concussion management and research, SLAM is widely acknowledged as one of sports neuropsychology's foundational paradigms (Webbe 2010).

The prominence of SLAM and its construction of "sport as laboratory" cements the logics of functionalism and the scientific experiment, including the value of quantitative measurement and statistical validity, as the dominant way of knowing and studying concussion. This notion extends into applications of the biopsychosocial model. Indeed, one of the perceived methodological strengths of the biopsychosocial model is how it enables researchers to isolate, control, and analyze the effects of multiple factors influencing concussion recovery (Wäljas et al. 2015). These formulations, however, reinforce conceptions of human beings as body machines organized according to quantifiable inputs and outputs that enable or disrupt healthy functioning (Stam 2000; Bendelow 2009). Such a compartmentalized approach to injury reproduces what scholars have identified as problematic philosophies underlying sports science and sports medicine, whereby athletes are imagined as well-tuned machines with doctors and scientists operating as highly skilled "technicians" responsible for the maintenance of the athletic body (Maguire 2011; Malcolm 2017).

This systematic approach to concussion extends to subjective psychosocial dimensions of concussion that are routinely quantified through standardized questionnaires and statistical analysis. For example, Step Two of the clinical office or off-field evaluation within the Sport Concussion Assessment Tool (SCAT), a widely used measurement tool, involves completing the Post-Concussion Symptom Scale in which athletes are instructed to rate their well-being on a Likert Scale from 0 to 6. The scale is further subdivided according to levels of severity, with 0 translating into "none" or no symptoms, 1 and 2 being classified as "mild," 3 and 4 as "moderate," and 5 and 6 as "severe." This questionnaire is made up of 22 categories ranging from physiological symptoms such as headache, neck pain, and blurred vision to emotional conditions such as "more emotional," "sadness," "irritability," and "nervous and anxious." The values for each category are then tabulated into a "symptom severity score" with a total possible score of 132. The popular Immediate Post-Concussion Assessment and Cognitive Testing (ImPACT) protocol includes a similar post-concussion symptom scale. These symptom checklists are typically administered alongside computerized tests assessing neuropsychological domains such as memory (verbal and visual), cognition, and reaction time (McCrory et al. 2017). Quantitative methodologies are also widely used to assess the influence of psychosocial factors such as athlete identities and personality traits on concussion recovery and reporting behaviors (O'Rourke et al. 2017; Kroshus et al. 2014).

These scales and tests, of course, are routinely validated to ensure that statistical measures are reliable and generalizable across multiple data sets (e.g., Allen and Gfeller 2011). There has also been great emphasis placed on ensuring that tests are properly interpreted by trained professionals and that athletes are unable to consciously manipulate test results (e.g., Erdal 2012; Echemendia et al. 2009). Yet it is harder to find studies that have gone as far as interrogating the "causal metaphysic" (Harré 2002) underpinning SLAM and its reliance on comparisons between healthy and injured populations. Such a logic presumes that baseline measurements document an "initial" state of well-being that is representative of an athlete's "normal" functioning and can serve as a reliable starting point from which future deviation can be assessed. Scholars have indeed questioned how the validity of quantitative health data often rests more broadly on the problematic assumption that variation in numerical scores directly coincides with impactful changes to a person's internal properties (Cromby 2007; Harré 2002). Some neuropsychologists acknowledge that the results of baseline tests might reflect and be confounded by the often transient nature of existing symptoms or even the day-to-day variability of an athlete's well-being (e.g., Asken et al. 2017). Yet these types of tests endure through medical databases as indicators of "true" pre-injury states even though they only record moments of experience frozen in time and decontextualized snapshots of athletes' lives.

Importantly, this formulation obscures not only the contextual specificities (i.e., personal histories and cultural environments but also enactments of gender, race, social class, sexuality, etc.) of an athlete's experience and the circumstances under which medical or scientific protocols are administered. Davidson (2016) explains that such faith in the capacity for clinicians to isolate and control aspects of the experience of brain injury "intensifies the illusion that selves operate atomistically, as singular, self-governing systems" (33). Such a functionalist view of concussion as a sum of component parts subtracts the individual from the meaningful social contexts in which they live, reducing complex life experiences to variables that can be readily modified through medical intervention. Acknowledging the limits of functionalism and quantification as means to capture the complexity of human experience, then, qualitative methods can offer distinct ways to account for the impact of social contexts in shaping concussion experiences.

Why Qualitative Research?

Promisingly, aligned with the spirit of the biopsychosocial model, the amount of qualitative work about concussion and TBI experiences is steadily growing within a research context dominated by quantitative methodologies. The bulk of qualitative research on this topic is comprised of psychological studies (Snell et al. 2017; Levack et al. 2010; Lininger et al. 2019; Tjong et al. 2017; Cusimano et al. 2016; Iadevaia et al. 2015; Moreau et al. 2014; Caron et al. 2017; Caron et al. 2013; Todd et al. 2018) and sociocultural analyses (Bridel et al. in this volume; Liston et al. 2016; Dean 2019; Cassilo and Sanderson 2018) that explore specific psychosocial aspects of TBI and concussion. These dimensions can include athlete attitudes, identities, emotions, social relationships, and cultural environments. Qualitative studies most often use interviews or focus groups to examine how athlete attitudes shape concussion (under)reporting behaviours or examine how athletes' lives change following concussion.

A primary focus of this qualitative work has been demonstrating how concussions disrupt notions of athletic identity and how the injury requires athletes to reconfigure their sense of self (Bridel et al. in this volume; Caron et al. 2013, 2017; Cusimano et al. 2016; Todd et al. 2018; Dean 2019; Moreau et al. 2014). Such studies are commendably attentive to how social norms and expectations around "what it means to be an athlete," such as playing through pain, self-sacrifice, and loyalty to a team, impact those living with concussions. Indeed, important scholarly work has been focused on how the occurrence and subsequent experiences of concussion are bound up with the celebration of a competitive, violent sporting masculinity through which displays of toughness are too frequently valorized as signs of manliness and commitment (Anderson and Kian 2012; Wiese-Bjornstal 2010; Cusimano et al. 2016; Dean 2019). Those aligned with the message of this scholarship have crafted concussion education programs encouraging athletes to resist impulses to play through a possible brain injury and instead seek appropriate medical attention.

Qualitative research can thus make important contributions to biopsychosocial conceptions of concussion by uncovering deep knowledge about psychosocial determinants that may slip through the cracks of quantitative scales and questionnaires. Still qualitative research is not in and of itself an escape from the limitations of the biopsychosocial model (Crossley 2008; Stam 2000). Indeed, it is not difficult to formulate qualitative research as a seemingly neutral mode of inquiry that reinforces rather than contests the causal metaphysic underlying quantitative analyses of health and illness. This point is especially evident within larger mixed methods studies, which tend to be structured around more traditional biomedical or statistical measures. In these instances, investigators often frame qualitative components as only providing opportunities to add nuance to quantitative findings or identify gaps in dominant statistical models. For example, if findings from quantitative surveys demonstrate that longer concussion recoveries were associated with athletes experiencing inadequate social support from family and friends, qualitative interviews may help identify reasons why this support failed to materialize for specific participants.

This example is consistent with Snell and colleagues' (2017, 1968) position that, "qualitative research can help explain factors underlying relationships observed in quantitative studies, interpret statistical relationships, and explore puzzling and inconsistent findings." Under such a framework, qualitative methods are typically relegated to a supporting role verifying or elaborating upon the primary (quantitative) findings. This supplementary relationship is organized according to principles of causal inference, with quantitative data identifying broad, generalizable trends and qualitative data providing examples of how these trends emerge in specific cases. These forms of "nested analysis" are commonly structured in such a way that quantitative aspects come first, with statistical findings shaping the directions of qualitative research conducted in secondary or "follow-up" phases. Yet these methodological structures reproduce problematic evidence hierarchies in which qualitative findings are presumed to only have value in relation to quantitative data, but seldom the other way around (Sommer Harrits 2011).

Yet qualitative findings can stand alone from or even contradict quantitative data, revealing the limits of statistical analysis or numerical models. Some concussion studies have indeed envisioned a more prominent role for qualitative methodologies that is not exclusively defined by the supremacy of quantitative measures. Tjong and colleagues (2017, 2) state that qualitative interviews can interrogate "unquantifiable concerns" shaping concussion experiences, whereas Caron and colleagues (2013, 169) write that "there is more to the concussion experience than what can be read from medical scans or physical symptoms." Such explanations position qualitative methods and subjective experience as providing knowledge otherwise inaccessible using quantitative techniques and statistical analyses. These justifications often highlight how qualitative methods offer a window into the "lived experience" of concussion, knowledge about which is best communicated in athletes' own words (e.g., Moreau et al. 2014; Bridel et al. in this volume).

Why Experience?

Important epistemological questions loom over qualitative studies of concussion: what do researchers believe they can learn from analyzing the "lived experience" of concussion? How do concussion experiences *become* evidence and for what purposes? These questions also reflect concerns from feminist scholars writing in the 1980s and 90s, whose collective work detailed the uses and limitations of experience as evidence. On the one hand, feminist standpoint theories promoted the value of women becoming their own theorists to reveal how intersecting inequitable social relations impacted their everyday lives. Other feminists, however, challenged the notion that "experiences" could stand alone as indisputable representations of a lived reality. In "The Evidence of Experience," Joan Scott (1991) problematizes the scholarly inclination to represent experience as incontrovertible "truth;" doing so, Scott argues, presumes there are natural and self-evident facets of existence, such as identity categories (e.g., "woman"), that each individual then experiences in their own way. Scott instead not only encourages us to confront the constructed nature of experience but foregrounds how socio-historical processes produce experiences and make certain experiences intelligible through language and cultural norms. In "Situated Knowledges," Donna Haraway (1988) similarly argues that "testimony from the position of oneself" is not an "innocent" representation of reality but is implicated in socio-historical *discursive* processes of meaning making and knowledge production. Thus, while athlete perspectives can importantly disrupt the pre-eminence of the scientific gaze in producing knowledge about concussion, it is crucial to avoid advancing athlete narratives as representing their own form of objectivity, envisioned as describing the reality of concussion rather than actively constructing a relationship between bodies, identities, and social worlds. Far from a foundational truth, then, "experience" is an effect of power and thus "is at once already an interpretation *and* something that needs to be interpreted" (Scott 1991, 97). Applied to concussion inquiries, qualitative research can center athletes' experiences but is most formidable in *explaining* how social norms and power relations shape experiences and the ways in which athletes communicate them.

Such epistemological tensions are evident in some qualitative concussion studies. Moreau et al.'s (2014, 73) study of American college athletes' lived experiences of concussion affirms, "it is assumed that the participants' responses were honest and accurate reflections of their lived experience and that they did not alter the responses to provide the socially acceptable or desired answer." This statement addresses the possibility that athletes could consciously manipulate their responses to satisfy the perceived expectations of the interviewers yet stops short of interrogating how the "socially acceptable or desired answer(s)" might be normalized across sports cultures and woven into athletes' interpretations of concussion experiences. Athletes' thought processes and understandings of their concussion experiences are not outside, and indeed are indelibly marked by, the language, norms, and values of the sports environments and social contexts in which they are situated. For example, an athlete may communicate that the worst part of their concussion was being unable to contribute to their team, and this account may accurately reflect how they felt throughout the duration of their injury. Yet this athlete's self-perceived disloyalty to their team (and why they felt inclined to highlight this aspect of their experience) is importantly shaped by cultural norms and expectations that encourage athletes to value their team's success over their own well-being.

Such concerns should especially guide analyses of the influence of athlete identity on concussion experiences. It is crucial that these types of investigations do not reify "athlete" as a self-evident identity category to which sports participants either conform or reject; rather, such studies should consider how "athlete" is not a natural category, but is instead continually shaped and reshaped by socio-historical forces and micro-level interactions (see Bridel et al. in this volume; Dean 2019; Todd et al. 2018). Therefore, while psychological programs for helping athletes manage disruptions to their identities represent valuable additions to individualized concussion treatment (e.g., Caron et al. 2013; Todd et al. 2018), it is similarly imperative that athlete norms are approached as potential sites of interrogation to help *prevent* such severe identity disruptions (Ventresca 2019).

Critical qualitative research also provides opportunities to explore how athlete experiences of concussion are impacted by biomedical actors and environments. While biopsychosocial studies are frequently attentive to how the quality of medical care or clinical tools shape concussion recoveries, it is less likely that such analyses interrogate how unpleasant experiences might be influenced by the very knowledge paradigms underlying concussion management strategies. Qualitative researchers have highlighted how TBI patients can become frustrated by interactions with doctors and clinicians (Caron et al. 2017; Davidson 2016; Shankar 2018). Autoethnographies written by Davidson (2016) and Shankar (2018) specifically explain how their experiences of TBI were adversely impacted by biomedical conceptions of injury and recovery, especially clinicians' over-reliance on quantitative modes of assessment. The authors recount how their experiential knowledge was routinely discounted in favor of "objective" measurements and how this disregard for their subjective knowledge provoked further psychological struggles throughout their recoveries. Not taking these narratives at face value, this autoethnographic work, is important in situating these experiences within broader socio-historical forces that privilege the authority of numbers across clinical settings, especially the illusion that objective measurements offer a "bird's-eye view" or "view from nowhere" insulated from social or historical influences (Haraway 1988). Davidson and Shankar's observations are linked to decades of science and technology studies (STS) research demonstrating how biomedical practices are indeed complex enactments of socio-historical conditions (e.g., Latour and Woolgar 1986; Jasanoff 2005; Haraway 1988).

Critical qualitative research can help map how clinical practices and scientific knowledge might similarly shape athletes' lived experiences of concussion. These scenarios can be sites to explore how quantitative metrics can exhibit agency and take on a life of their own, not merely describing their objects of study but actively pushing and pulling human lives into shapes molded through dominant knowledge paradigms (Pitts-Taylor 2016; Mol 2002). Research into psychosocial dimensions of concussion would be well served by documenting how athletes navigate tensions between their own embodied knowledge and institutionalized expertise from clinicians and scientists built through the veneration of quantitative metrics. Doing so could contextualize how, for example, athletes resolve contradictions between subjective knowledge of their recovery and quantitative measures representing their progress (or lack thereof) in the context of structured return-to-play protocols. Such studies could delve further into epistemological conflicts whereby scientific knowledge about concussion is widely characterized as "uncertain," yet clinicians still tend to marginalize athletes' experiential embodied knowledge by appealing to the authority of scientific knowledge (Malcolm 2017). Critically examining how athletes engage with scientific knowledge and navigate their clinical experiences would importantly disrupt the conception of science and biomedicine as "neutral," "objective" tools within the biopsychosocial model (Stam 2000). Instead, qualitative studies could explain, first, how clinical practices including numeric scales have tangible (positive and/or negative) consequences on biological, psychological, and social dimensions of an athletes' recovery; and second, such research could reveal how clinical concussion management and return-to-play protocols are themselves subject to socio-historical processes shaping their impacts on athlete experiences.

In sum, while it is encouraging that qualitative research into athletes' lived experiences of concussion is increasingly appearing alongside quantitative components of the biopsychosocial model, these studies must actively contextualize athlete experiences as produced in and through a specific set of socio-historical processes. Such analysis will allow inquiries into how athletes interpret their experiences of concussion as well as provide insight into what values and norms enable and constrain these interpretations. Yet, importantly, it is necessary for concussion researchers to careful theorize how they integrate qualitative knowledge alongside the quantitative paradigms largely defining the biopsychosocial model. Specifically, researchers cannot ignore tensions across these ways of knowing; facilitating quantification through the compartmentalization of concussion experiences into discrete variables can indeed clash with what qualitative research reveals about the co-production of the often indivisible dimensions of experience.

Is Functionalism a Fatal Flaw?

In their report on future directions for sports concussion assessment and management, McCrea et al. (2015) acknowledge that it is difficult for individual studies to incorporate the broad scope of outcomes falling under the umbrella of the biopsychosocial model. The authors admit that, because of these challenges, "a fully integrated model has not yet been achieved" (278). Yet the reliance on compartmentalized measurement of separate variables presents additional challenges for the model's design as an "integrated" approach to concussion. That is, the model is predicated on the reciprocal "interplay" or "interaction" of biological, psychological, and social factors; yet since Engel's initial formulation, there has been little clarification around how the biopsychosocial model conceptualizes the nature of such interactions (Stam 2000; Crossley 2008; Bendelow 2009). Critics have noted that, despite the promise of an integrated framework for understanding the interplay of multiple factors, the biopsychosocial model facilitates a further fragmentation of human experiences. Biopsychosocial approaches to concussion evaluation perpetuate this problem through their indebtedness to SLAM and the broader logics of functionalism.

The need for more integrative models is especially noticeable in biopsychosocial conceptions of the emotional experiences of concussion, including clinically diagnosed depression and anxiety disorders. The primary question I have encountered across the literature on the emotional or psychiatric aspects of concussion relates to the extent to which these symptoms are directly induced by brain trauma. As Solomon and colleagues (2016) explain, while depressive symptoms "may be an acute result and neurophysiological response to the concussive event itself, it may also be due to other reasons, such as frustrations of being withheld from play or other psychosocial factors" (15). Harmon and colleagues (2013) similarly write that it is difficult to determine which psychiatric disturbances "preceded the concussion, which have been caused by the concussion, and which symptoms are worsened after the concussion" (5).

Importantly, neuropsychological studies have also identified pre-injury depression or anxiety (or histories of mental health diagnoses) as key predictors for determining which athletes are most at risk of prolonged recoveries from concussion (Yang et al. 2015; Iverson et al. 2017; Solomon et al. 2016; Bloom et al. 2004). However, any causal relationship between brain trauma and emotional disturbances are also confounded by psychology research suggesting that athletes with musculoskeletal injuries also experience strong emotional reactions in line with those who have sustained concussions (Mainwaring et al. 2010). If emotional disturbances can accompany sports injuries beyond the brain, then it is conceivable that emotionally fraught concussion recoveries are precipitated more by the psychosocial dimensions of injuries in general rather than the neuropsychological specifics of brain trauma.

The magnitude of these research directions around emotions is immense: evidence that post-concussion psychiatric symptoms are more a result of psychosocial determinants than neurophysiological damage raises questions about whether the psychological effects of concussion are demonstrably different or more severe than other types of sports injuries. Proposed conclusions within these debates are implicated in a contentious research climate whereby scientists and advocates hold up emotional distress from concussion as evidence for the injury's distinctiveness and severity; yet, conversely, other scientists and clinicians are suspicious of what they believe is linear thinking positioning "concussions or subconcussive impacts as the cause of all neuropsychiatric ills" (Solomon 2018, 303). The perceived capacity to isolate psychosocial from neuropathological components of concussion will fuel further skepticism around whether symptoms are specific to brain injury or simply manifestations of other physiological or psychological concerns (e.g., Asken et al. 2017). Conclusions about the origins of psychosocial aspects of concussion are perhaps most noticeably informing heated debates about the perceived links between brain trauma, depression, and athlete suicide (e.g., Iverson 2014). Methodologically, these conversations also embolden claims that future advancements in neuroimaging will facilitate more definitive distinctions between psychosocial and neurophysiological sources of concussion symptoms (McCuddy et al. 2018; Ho et al. 2018).

Yet the very proposition of studying biological and emotional effects of concussion in isolation presupposes that these experiences can be neatly separated in the first place. The methodological decisions and conclusions coming out of these mostly neuroscientific research directions reproduce a compartmentalized mental versus physical health dichotomy, which has been highlighted in critiques of the biopsychosocial model (Bendelow 2009). Such a critique has been especially powerful in challenging dominant conceptions of pain and pain management. Biopsychosocial approaches to pain management are reductionistic, troubled by the inseparable experiences of pain as emotion and pain as physical sensation. The compartmentalized biopsychosocial model is further confounded by the ontological and temporal complexities of pain and the inability for scientific methods to determine whether emotion is a cause, component, or consequence of pain (or all three at once) (Bendelow and Williams 1995; Lima, Alves, and Turato 2014). Reducing pain to the realm of biology means that its origins should be readily located somewhere in the body and captured through objective measurement of biological variables; yet pain is only intelligible through subjective experience and an individual's expression of a state of well-being (often codified through biopsychosocial numerical scales designed to measure severity). How a patient articulates their feelings of pain is influenced not only by degrees of neural activity, but also their emotions and personal histories, as well as social norms and the cultural context in which the assessment occurs. In sport environments, norms associating playing through injury with masculine toughness and grit shape how athletes embody and describe pain, but these experiences are also influenced by expectations underlying interactions between athletes, coaches, and medical professionals (Safai 2003; Malcolm 2009).

Researchers interested in the complexities of concussion should take important lessons from these observations about the multiple concurrent materializations of pain. Whereas the biopsychosocial model creates important space for emotions and psychiatric disturbances (and their relations to psychosocial factors) to be taken seriously as part of the diagnostic picture of concussion, dominant methods still tend to objectify emotional experiences as "things" that can be isolated, quantified, and treated as ontologically distinct from the biological symptoms of concussion. Rather than conceptualizing psychosocial elements of concussion as contextually situated and embodied processes, current applications of the biopsychosocial model often position these experiences as static, universal variables within measurable cause-and-effect trajectories (Cromby 2007). It is worth exploring, therefore, how studies of concussion might benefit from a "non-objectifying view of emotion as relational flows, fluxes or currents in-between people and places, rather than 'things' or 'objects' to be studied" (Bondi, Davidson, and Smith 2005, 3). Qualitative methods are well-suited to explore the complexities of emotion and its embodiments. Yet, again, it is unclear how such methods could be adequately incorporated into the compartmentalized biopsychosocial model when the knowledge they produce often challenges the logics of functionalist paradigms.

Critical qualitative concussion research can actively resist the objectification of emotions if these studies support shifts in thinking about how the multiple dimensions of injury materialize *together* through embodied experience. This notion is exemplified by former college quarterback Casey Cochran's (2016) account of the immediate aftermath of a concussion in *The Players' Tribune*,

> "The only word I know to describe the first few moments after a concussion is limbo—there are a few moments between the world that you

were just a part of and your new brain-injured reality. When I regained consciousness, I knew I was on the ground. My head was seized with tremendous pressure, and that same awful, familiar depression from previous head injuries came over me—like a dark, heavy blanket, swallowing me up."

Cochran's portrayal does not need to be taken as providing irrefutable "truth" about the temporal sequence through which symptoms materialized following impact; rather, his story highlights the existential messiness of his experience and how extreme physical sensations, intense emotions, and memories instantaneously flooded his consciousness as he lay on the ground. The descriptive depth of Cochran's account reinforces how emotional aspects of concussion are non-linear and unpredictable, informed by personal histories, and co-constructed with biological sensations. How Cochran describes the confusion and unruliness characterizing his experience vividly contrasts the ontological orderliness projected onto concussion through the biopsychosocial model. Indeed, his depiction illustrates the power of narrative as an alternative way of representing concussion that defies attempts to compartmentalize injury according to separate categories of experience.

The biopsychosocial model, through its very structure, makes claims about what a concussion *is*: an injury constituted through the *interaction* of biological, psychological, and social components. Following Keller (2000), however, conceptualizing concussion as an "interaction" between body, mind, and environment positions each domain as intrinsically distinct, and separately functioning, parts of a broader bodily system. Thus, despite the well-used imagery of "overlap" and "interplay" of different dimensions of experience, proponents of the biopsychosocial models fail to reconcile the philosophical implications of such language with the model's commitments to functionalism. How can dimensions of experience emerge together yet be systematically broken apart for the purposes of scientific study? This type of compartmentalization furthers the illusion that clinicians and researchers, by isolating components of concussion, can theoretically create empty space *between* biological, psychological, and social components of human life. This, I believe, is an irreconcilable flaw of the biopsychosocial model's reliance on functionalism; as Keller (2000, 30) writes, "the image of separable ingredients continues to exert a surprisingly strong hold on our imagination, even long after we have learned better." The limitations of functionalist ways of knowing illustrate the importance of acknowledging the inherent limits of the biopsychosocial model and exploring new modes of conceptualizing concussion as a human experience.

Beyond the Biopsychosocial

Throughout this chapter, I have outlined how the biopsychosocial model further entrenches a compartmentalized approach to understanding concussion that in turn supports the construction of quantifiable, causal trajectories between the biological, psychological, and social dimensions of injury. I have similarly argued that, while the model certainly opens up space for exploring the psychological and social aspects of concussion, it also constrains how knowledge about these dimensions gets produced. As the biopsychosocial model organizes experiences of concussion into discrete categories, it falls short of providing a truly integrated *biopsychosocial* framework, and instead conceptualizes concussion as biological *and* psychological *and* social. Here, the conjunction "and" signifies how the model reproduces the illusion that scientific techniques can dissect experience into "separable ingredients" that can be analyzed in isolation from each other. Such a compartmentalized view of concussion cannot account for how human experiences are constituted through an amalgam of embodied and cultural processes that continuously shape one another and therefore cannot be separated as distinct entities (Keller 2000). While attention to these concerns may be implicitly informing researchers' conclusions and methodological decisions, these deliberations need to be open, public conversations that also incorporate critical perspectives from disciplines beyond those already accepted as dominant contributors to biopsychosocial theorizing.

Feminist science and technology studies scholars have crafted theories that could serve as alternatives to the biopsychosocial model, providing more integrated formulations of how the biological, psychological, and social are in uninterrupted dialogue with one another. Samantha Frost (2016) uses the term *biocultural* to encapsulate the mutual constitution of body and environment. Frost emphasizes that "biocultural" is meant to draw attention to how the organic constitution and personhood of human beings is made through continuous interrelation with the worlds we inhabit. The notion of biocultural, then, resists a vision of human beings as self-contained entities with bodies that can be (even theoretically) isolated or disconnected from the material, social, and symbolic processes of "culture." Victoria Pitts-Taylor's (2016) theorization of the *biosocial* similarly stresses that the biological body is not solely representative of nature or culture but is "a specific configuration of matter and meaning that achieves itself in entanglement with the world" (35). She argues that biological matter is inherently relational, inseparable from the organic and social organizations of its surroundings. Both Frost and Pitts-Taylor deny the existence of fixed boundaries between the body and material and social environments, and instead propose dynamic, open exchanges between biological and social dimensions of human life. Drawing from feminist new materialism traditions, these theorists propose that the body and environment should not be viewed as distinct entities with identifiable influences on the other; rather, the biological *is always* social and the social *is always* biological.

Such an ontological shift would radically reconfigure conceptions of concussion and how individuals experience the injury as a lived, embodied phenomenon. I end this chapter with a call for additional critical reflection about how current configurations of the biopsychosocial model confine the unwieldly, volatile experience of concussion through predictable, controllable knowledge practices. My analysis highlights the need to unsettle the current epistemological dominance of controlled quantifiable experiments in concussion research that fail to adequately represent the messy, fluid co-construction of biological, psychological, and social aspects of injury. Any new paradigm, however, should re-center critical qualitative modes of inquiry not only in thoroughly contextualizing and interpreting athlete experiences, but also in refining the philosophical foundations of concussion research.

Yet this proposal is not meant to entirely denounce the merits of quantitative methods or contributions of the life sciences in building nuanced, socially situated conceptions of concussion. Far from a rallying cry for disciplinary antagonism, this chapter follows scholars who have identified much promise for collaboration across the social and life sciences for more complex conceptions of human experience (Choudhary et al. 2009; Pitts-Taylor 2016). Capturing the co-constitution of the biological and social through methodological and clinical practices will certainly require substantial interdisciplinary theorizing about the synergy between the "nature"—and "culture"—of concussion experiences. Many science and technology studies scholars have identified the social entanglements of neuroscience and the brain as potential sites for fruitful collaboration across different ways of knowing; yet analyses of the self as embodied and neurobiology as social have largely remained peripheral to concussion research, especially in sports contexts. Critical qualitative research, then, can introduce possibilities for mapping and refining the intricacies of biomedical and scientific processes that define how we know and understand concussion and TBI. Questioning underlying assumptions in this way can be done in the interest of enhancing the methodological rigour of concussion studies while also acknowledging the complex interrelations of bodies, experiences, and sites of knowledge production.

References

Allen, Brittany J., and Jeffrey D. Gfeller. 2011. "The Immediate Post-Concussion Assessment and Cognitive Testing Battery and Traditional Neuropsychological Measures: A Construct and Concurrent Validity Study." *Brain Injury* 25 (2): 179–191.

Anderson, Eric, and Edward M. Kian. 2012. "Examining Media Contestation of Masculinity and Head Trauma in the National Football League." *Men and Masculinities* 15 (2): 152–173.

Asken, Breton M., Aliyah R. Snyder, M. Seth Smith, Jason L. Zaremski, and Russell M. Bauer. 2017. "Concussion-like Symptom Reporting in Non-Concussed Adolescent Athletes." *Clinical Neuropsychologist* 31 (1): 138–153.

Barth, Jeffrey T., Daniel J. Harvey, Jason R. Freeman, and Donna K. Broshek. 2010. "Sports as Laboratory Assessment Model." In *Handbook of Sport Neuropsychology*, edited by Frank M Webbe, 75–90. New York: Springer Publishing Company.

Bendelow, Gillian. 2009. *Health, Emotion, and the Body.* Malden, MA: Polity Press.

Bendelow, Gillian, and Simon J. Williams. 1995. "Transcending the Dualisms: Towards a Sociology of Pain." *Sociology of Health and Illness* 17 (2): 139–165.

Bloom, Gordon A., Amanda S. Horton, Paul McCrory, and Karen M. Johnston. 2004. "Sport Psychology and Concussion: New Impacts to Explore." *British Journal of Sports Medicine* 38 (5): 519. https://doi.org/10.1136/bjsm.2004.011999.

Bondi, Liz, Joyce Davidson, and Mick Smith. 2005. "Introduction: Geography's 'Emotional Turn.'" In *Emotional Geographies*, edited by Joyce Davidson, Liz Bondi, and Mick Smith, 1–16. New York: Routledge.

Caron, Jeffrey G., Gordon A. Bloom, Karen M. Johnston, and Catherine Sabiston. 2013. "Effects of Multiple Concussions on Retired National Hockey League Players." *Journal of Sport & Exercise Psychology* 35.

Caron, Jeffrey G., Lee Schaefer, Daphnée André-Morin, and Shawn Wilkinson. 2017. "A Narrative Inquiry into a Female Athlete's Experiences with Protracted Concussion Symptoms." *International Perspectives on Stress & Coping* 22 (6): 501–513.

Cassilo, David, and Jimmy Sanderson. 2018. "From Social Isolation to Becoming an Advocate: Exploring Athletes' Grief Discourse About Lived Concussion Experiences in Online Forums." *Communication & Sport*, July. doi:10.1177/2167479518790039.

Choudhary, Suparna, Saskia Kathi Nagel, and Jan Slaby. 2009. "Critical Neuroscience: Linking Neuroscience and Society Through Critical Practice." *BioSocieties* 4 (1): 61–77.

Cochran, Casey. 2016. "13 Concussions." *The Players' Tribune*, July 5. www.theplayerstribune.com/casey-cochran-uconn-football-concussions/.

Cromby, John. 2007. "Integrating Social Science with Neuroscience: Potentials and Problems." *BioSocieties* 2 (2): 149–169.

Crossley, Michelle. 2008. "Critical Health Psychology: Developing and Refining the Approach." *Social and Personality Psychology Compass* 2 (1): 21–33.

Cusimano, Michael, Jane Topolovec-Vranic, Stanley Zhang, Sarah J. Mullen, Matthew Wong, and Gabriela Ilie. 2016. "Factors Influencing the Underreporting of Concussion in Sports: A Qualitative Study of Minor Hockey Participants." *Clinical Journal of Sport Medicine* 27.

Davidson, Joyce. 2016. "Plenary Address—A Year of Living 'Dangerously': Reflections on Risk, Trust, Trauma and Change." *Emotion, Space and Society* 18: 28–34.

Dean, Nikolaus A. 2019. "'Just Act Normal': Concussion and the (Re)Negotiation of Athletic Identity." *Sociology of Sport Journal* 36 (1): 22–31.

Echemendia, Ruben J., Sally E. Herring, and Julian Bailes. 2009. "Who Should Conduct and Interpret the Neuropsychological Assessment in Sports-Related Concussion?" *British Journal of Sports Medicine* 43 (Supplement 1): i32–i35.

Echemendia, Ruben J., and Laura J. Julian. 2001. "Mild Traumatic Brain Injury in Sports: Neuropsychology's Contribution to a Developing Field." *Neuropsychology Review* 11 (2): 69–88.

Engel, George L. 1977. "The Need for a New Medical Model: A Challenge for Biomedicine." *Science* 196 (4286): 129–136.

Erdal, Kristi. 2012. "Neuropsychological Testing for Sports-Related Concussion: How Athletes Can Sandbag Their Baseline Testing Without Detection." *Archives of Clinical Neuropsychology* 27 (5): 473–479.

Frost, Samantha. 2016. *Biocultural Creatres: Toward a New Theory of the Human.* Durham, NC: Duke University Press.

Haraway, Donna. 1988. "Situated Knowledges: The Science Question in Feminism and the Privilege of Partial Perspective." *Feminist Studies* 14 (3): 575–599.

Harré, Rom. 2002. "Material Objects in Social Worlds." *Theory, Culture & Society* 19 (5–6): 23–33.

Ho, Rachelle A., Geoffrey B. Hall, Michael D. Noseworthy, and Carol DeMatteo. 2018. "An Emotional Go/No-Go FMRI Study in Adolescents with Depressive Symptoms Following Concussion." *International Journal of Psychophysiology* 132: 62–73.

Iadevaia, Cheree, Trevor Roiger, and Mary Beth Zwart. 2015. "Qualitative Examination of Adolescent Health-Related Quality of Life at 1 Year Postconcussion." *Journal of Athletic Training* 50 (11): 1182–1189.

Iverson, Grant L. 2012. "A Biopsychosocial Conceptualization of Poor Outcome from Mild Traumatic Brain Injury." In *PTSD and Mild Traumatic Brain Injury,* edited by Jennifer J. Vasterling, Richard A. Bryant, and Terence M. Keane. New York: The Guilford Press.

Iverson, Grant L. 2014. "Chronic Traumatic Encephalopathy and Risk of Suicide in Former Athletes." *British Journal of Sports Medicine* 48 (2): 162 LP–164 LP.

Iverson, Grant L., Andrew J. Gardner, Douglas P. Terry, Jennie L. Ponsford, Allen K. Sills, Donna K. Broshek, and Gary S. Solomon. 2017. "Predictors of Clinical Recovery from Concussion: A Systematic Review." *British Journal of Sports Medicine* 51 (12): 941–948.

Jasanoff, Sheila. 2005. *Designs on Nature: Science and Democracy in Europe and the United States.* Princeton: Princeton University Press.

Keller, Evelyn Fox. 2000. *The Century of the Gene.* Cambridge, MA: Harvard University Press.

Kroshus, Emily, Christine M. Baugh, Daniel H. Daneshvar, and Kasisomayajula Viswanath. 2014. "Understanding Concussion Reporting Using a Model Based on the Theory of Planned Behavior." *Journal of Adolescent Health* 54 (3): 269–274.

Latour, Bruno, and Steve Woolgar. 1986. *Laboratory Life: The Construction of Scientific Facts.* Princeton: Princeton University Press.

Levack, William M.M., Nicola M. Kayes, and Joanna K. Fadyl. 2010. "Experience of Recovery and Outcome Following Traumatic Brain Injury: A Metasynthesis of Qualitative Research." *Disability and Rehabilitation* 32 (12): 986–999.

Lima, Daniela Dantas, Vera Lucia Pereira Alves, and Egberto Ribeiro Turato. 2014. "The Phenomenological-Existential Comprehension of Chronic Pain: Going Beyond the Standing Healthcare Models." *Philosophy, Ethics, and Humanities in Medicine* 9 (2): 1–10.

Lininger, Monica R., Heidi A. Wayment, Debbie I. Craig, Ann Hergatt Huffman, and Taylor S. Lane. 2019. "Improving Concussion-Reporting Behavior in National Collegiate Athletic Association Division I Football Players: Evidence for the Applicability of the Socioecological Model for Athletic Trainers." *Journal of Athletic Training* 54 (1): 21–29.

Liston, Katie, Mark McDowell, Dominic Malcolm, Andrea Scott-Bell, and Ivan Waddington. 2016. "On Being 'Head Strong': The Pain Zone and Concussion in Non-Elite Rugby Union." *International Review for the Sociology of Sport,* December. doi:1012690216679966.

Maguire, Joseph A. 2011. "Human Sciences, Sports Sciences and the Need to Study People 'in the Round'." *Sport in Society* 14 (7–8): 898–912.

Mainwaring, Lynda M., Michael Hutchison, Sean M. Bisschop, Paul Comper, and Doug W. Richards. 2010. "Emotional Response to Sport Concussion Compared to ACL Injury." *Brain Injury* 24 (4): 589–597.

Malcolm, Dominic. 2009. "Medical Uncertainty and Clinician—Athlete Relations: The Management of Concussion Injuries in Rugby Union." *Sociology of Sport Journal* 26: 191–210.

Malcolm, Dominic. 2017. *Sport, Medicine, and Health: The Medicalization of Sport?* London: Routledge.

McCrea, Michael, Donna K. Broshek, and Jeffrey T. Barth. 2015. "Sports Concussion Assessment and Management: Future Research Directions." *Brain Injury* 29 (2): 276–282.

McCrory, Paul, Willem Meeuwisse, Jiří Dvorak, Mark Aubry, Julian Bailes, Steven Broglio, Robert C Cantu, et al. 2017. "Consensus Statement on Concussion in Sport—the 5 Th International Conference on Concussion in Sport Held in Berlin, October 2016." *British Journal of Sports Medicine* 51 (11): 1–10.

McCuddy, William T., Lezlie Y. España, Lindsay D. Nelson, Rasmus M. Birn, Andrew R. Mayer, and Timothy B. Meier. 2018. "Association of Acute Depressive Symptoms and Functional Connectivity of Emotional Processing Regions Following Sport-Related Concussion." *NeuroImage: Clinical* 19: 434–442.

Mol, Annemarie. 2002. *The Body Multiple: Ontology in Medical Practice*. Durham, NC: Duke University Press.

Moreau, Matthew S., Jody Langdon, and Thomas A. Buckley. 2014. "The Lived Experience of an In-Season Concussion Amongst NCAA Division I Student-Athletes." *International Journal of Exercise Science* 7 (1): 62–74.

O'Rourke, Daniel J., Ronald E. Smith, Stephanie Punt, David B. Coppel, and David Breiger. 2017. "Psychosocial Correlates of Young Athletes' Self-Reported Concussion Symptoms During the Course of Recovery." *Sport, Exercise, and Performance Psychology* 6 (3): 262–276.

Panczykowski, D.M., and J.E. Pardini. 2014. "The Multidisciplinary Concussion Management Program." *Progress in Neurological Surgery* 28: 195–212.

Pitts-Taylor, Victoria. 2016. *The Brain's Body: Neuroscience and Corporeal Politics*. Durham, NC: Duke University Press.

Safai, Parissa. 2003. "Healing the Body in the 'Culture of Risk': Examining the Negotiation of Treatment Between Sport Medicine Clinicians and Injured Athletes in Canadian Intercollegiate Sport." *Sociology of Sport Journal* 20 (2): 127–146.

Scott, Joan W. 1991. "The Evidence of Experience." *Critical Inquiry* 17 (4): 773–797.

Shankar, Sneha. 2018. "An Auto-Ethnography About Recovering Awareness Following Brain Injury: Is My Truth Valid?" *Qualitative Inquiry* 24 (1): 56–69.

Silverberg, Noah D., Andrew J. Gardner, Jeffrey R. Brubacher, William J. Panenka, Jun Jian Li, and Grant L. Iverson. 2015. "Systematic Review of Multivariable Prognostic Models for Mild Traumatic Brain Injury." *Journal of Neurotrauma* 526: 517–526.

Smith, Joan. 1975. "The Failure of Functionalism." *Philosophy of the Social Sciences* 5 (1): 33–42.

Snell, Deborah L., Rachelle Martin, Lois J. Surgenor, Richard J. Siegert, and E. Jean C. Hay-Smith. 2017. "What's Wrong with Me? Seeking a Coherent

Understanding of Recovery after Mild Traumatic Brain Injury." *Disability and Rehabilitation* 39 (19): 1968–1975.

Solomon, Gary S., Andrew W. Kuhn, and Scott L. Zuckerman. 2016. "Depression as a Modifying Factor in Sport-Related Concussion: A Critical Review of the Literature." *The Physician and Sportsmedicine* 44 (1): 14–19.

Solomon, Gary. 2018. "Chronic Traumatic Encephalopathy in Sports: A Historical and Narrative Review. *Developmental Neuropsychology* 43 (4): 279–311.

Sommer Harrits, Gitte. 2011. "More Than Method?: A Discussion of Paradigm Differences Within Mixed Methods Research." *Journal of Mixed Methods Research* 5 (2): 150–166.

Stam, Henderikus J. 2000. "Theorizing Health and Illness: Functionalism, Subjectivity and Reflexivity." *Journal of Health Psychology* 5 (3): 273–283.

Tjong, Vehniah K., Hayden P. Baker, Charles J. Cogan, Melissa Montoya, Tory R. Lindley, and Michael A. Terry. 2017. "Concussions in NCAA Varsity Football Athletes: A Qualitative Investigation of Player Perception and Return to Sport." *Journal of the American Academy of Orthopaedic Surgeons. Global Research & Reviews* 1 (8): e070.

Todd, Ryan, Shree Bhalerao, Michael T. Vu, Sophie Soklaridis, and Michael D. Cusimano. 2018. "Understanding the Psychiatric Effects of Concussion on Constructed Identity in Hockey Players: Implications for Health Professionals." *PLOS One* 13 (2): e0192125.

Ventresca, Matt. 2019. "The Curious Case of CTE: Mediating Materialities of Traumatic Brain Injury." *Communication & Sport* 7 (2): 135–156. https://doi.org/10.1177/2167479518761636.

Ventresca, Matt. 2020. "The Tangled Multiplicities of CTE: Scientific Uncertainty and the Infrastructures of Traumatic Brain Injury." In *Sports, Society, and Technology: Bodies, Practices, and Knowledge Production*, edited by Jennifer Sterling, and Mary G. McDonald. New York: Palgrave Macmillan.

Vidal, Fernando, and Francisco Ortega. 2011. "Approaching the Neurocultural Spectrum: An Introduction." In *NeuroCultures: Glimpses into an Expanding Universe*, edited by Francisco Ortega, and Fernando Vidal, 7–28. New York: Peter Lang.

Wäljas, Minna, Grant L. Iverson, Rael T. Lange, Ullamari Hakulinen, Prasun Dastidar, Heini Huhtala, Suvi Liimatainen, Kaisa Hartikainen, and Juha Öhman. 2015. "A Prospective Biopsychosocial Study of the Persistent Post-Concussion Symptoms Following Mild Traumatic Brain Injury." *Journal of Neurotrauma* 32 (8): 534–547.

Webbe, Frank M. 2010. "Introduction to Sport Neuropsychology." In *The Handbook of Sport Neuropsychology*, edited by Frank M Webbe, 1–16. New York: Springer Publishing Company.

Wiese-Bjornstal, Diane M. 2010. "Psychology and Socioculture Affect Injury Risk, Response, and Recovery in High-Intensity Athletes: A Consensus Statement." *Scandanavian Journal of Medicine & Science in Sports* 20 (2): 103–111.

Yang, Jingzhen, Corinne Peek-asa, Tracey Covassin, James C. Torner, Jingzhen Yang, Corinne Peek-asa, Tracey Covassin, James C. Torner, and Corinne Peek-asa. 2015. "Post-Concussion Symptoms of Depression and Anxiety in Division I Collegiate Athletes." *Developmental Neuropsychology* 40 (1): 18–23.

Index

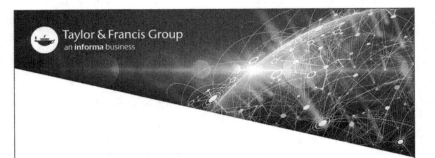

Printed in the United States
by Baker & Taylor Publisher Services